STOP BEING FAT

Lose The BS, Lose The Weight

Written by Author
Donna Phelan

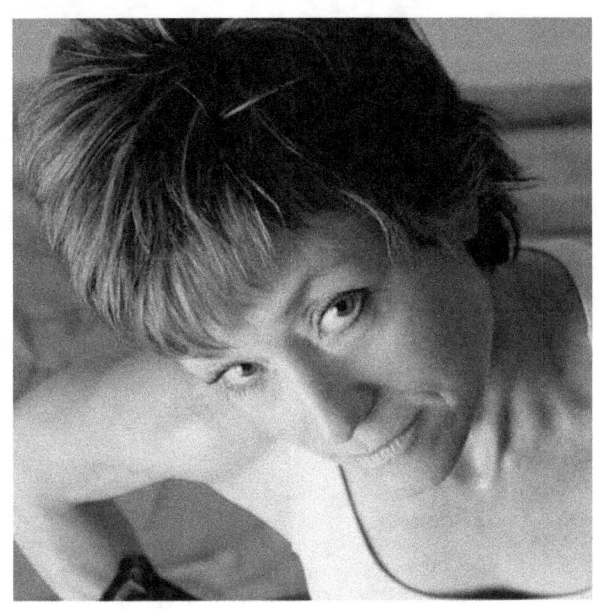

Author

Donna Phelan

Donna Phelan is an ACE (American Council on Exercise) certified Group Fitness Instructor and co-owner of KnowSweat Workouts in Indianapolis, IN. She is also a monthly contributor and columnist at Health Minute Magazine www.HealthMinuteMagazine.com. Overweight all through childhood and her teenage years, Donna lost 87 pounds at the age of 19 and has successfully maintained her weight and fitness for over 35 years. Donna uses her real life experience with losing and maintaining her weight to educate and motivate her clients through the Stop Being Fat Network at KnowSweat Workouts. Donna welcomes reader comments at Donna@StopBeingFat101.com.

Dedication

I want to thank all the special people in my life who, by their love and caring, inspire me to be the best I can be for them.

Disclaimer and Terms of Use

Disclaimer and Terms of Use: No information contained in this book should be considered as physical, health related, financial, tax or legal advise. Your reliance upon information and content obtained by you at or through this publication is solely at your own risk. The author assumes no liability or responsibility for damage or injury to you, other persons, or property arising from any use of any product, information, idea, or instruction contained in the content provided to you through this book.

Contents

Prologue

If you are reading this book, it is likely that you are fat. Not only are you fat, but you are unhappy with your fatness. There is joy in your life, to be sure – friends and family that love you, fond memories and wonderful experiences. But, you are the only one who knows how you feel when you struggle into a narrow theater seat, hand over your credit card to purchase clothing in a bigger size, or overhear the hurtful comments of strangers.

In the pages that follow, you won't learn the secret to weight loss...there isn't one. I'm not going to reveal the best diet...they all work if you follow them. Don't expect my number one exercise for burning fat, a list of the 10 best foods to boost metabolism, or the sneaky environmental conditions that are causing you to gain weight. The principle of weight loss is incredibly simple. It does not require you to buy anything from me except the truth. Sounds easy enough, but the emotional journey can be quite painful for those who have been searching to blame anyone or anything but themselves.

Life is a story. Up to this point, your story has been one of blaming your environment, blaming others, and looking for the quick and easy fix to your unhappiness.

Take a moment and think of your favorite book, one that you read cover to cover in record time, one that you raved about and eagerly loaned to your friends just so you could share it with someone. Have you got one in mind? When you read that book – the BEST book ever! – you never once regretted finishing a chapter and starting the next chapter. In fact, you looked forward to the next chapter...and the next chapter, savoring every word.

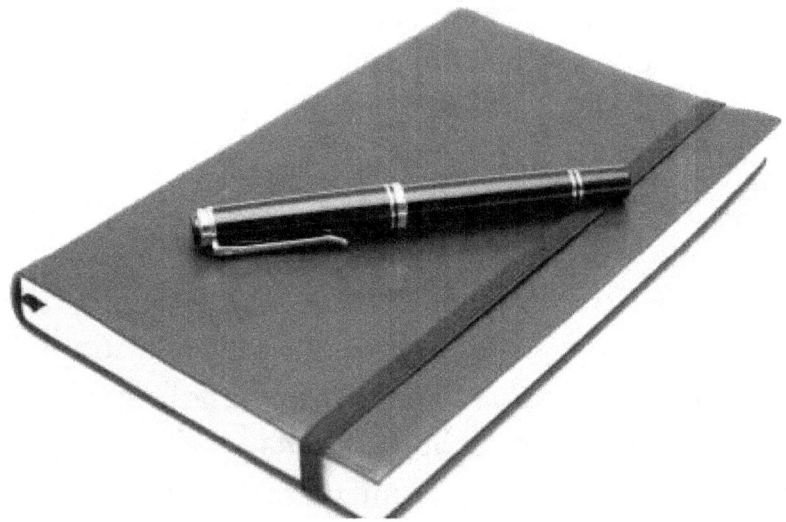

As the main character in your own story, it is time to start writing again, to turn the page on a new chapter. Why do you relive the same chapter over and over, never moving on, continuing to be the same fat person, living the same fat life? As Albert Einstein said, the definition of insanity is doing the same thing over and over again and expecting different results. It is time to stop playing the fat character and create a new thin character. The thin character is a **completely** different person living a **completely** different life, not the old fat character who makes minor changes in the hopes that weight loss and fitness will 'happen.' To continue to relive the same chapter is to continue to stay fat.   If you want a new chapter, start writing it! YOU are the only one who can!

If you are fat, and completely happy with yourself, this book is not for you. It is not my place to tell you to change, nor should you allow anyone to do so.   If you are among the smallest percentage of the population with a medical condition that inhibits your weight loss, this book is not for you. Seek the advice of a medical professional. But, if you are fat and not happy with the fat you, this book is like no other weight loss advice, gadget or gimmick you have ever tried. It is not my purpose to convince fat people to lose weight. My goal is to motivate those who want to lose fat by revealing the truth about their lives, their feelings and the changes required to start a new chapter.

So, if you are ready to Stop Being Fat, turn the page.....

1

How Can YOU Lose Weight?

The answer is that <u>YOU</u> cannot!

The principle of weight loss is incredibly simple: take in fewer calories than you burn, and you WILL lose weight. It can't fail! Simple in principle; difficult in execution. Why is it so difficult?

There are thousands of diet programs and books available to choose from and a gym on every corner. You can find the answer to any question regarding nutrition or exercise 24/7 on the internet from the comfort of your keyboard. How is it possible that you, and America, and the world are getting fatter and fatter? Clearly, whatever we are doing, however we are attacking the problem, it isn't working.

Most people focus on the wrong thing. What diet should I follow? What's the best exercise? If you have tried to lose weight unsuccessfully, you are like most fat people – about 90% fail. And, like most fat individuals, you have failed more than once. You have no doubt tried a variety of diets, and just as many gyms or workout programs. Of course, diet and exercise are key in weight loss. But, any diet works if you follow it, any exercise burns calories if you perform it. If you are honest enough to examine this a bit more closely, you will see that the one common denominator in all this failure is YOU.

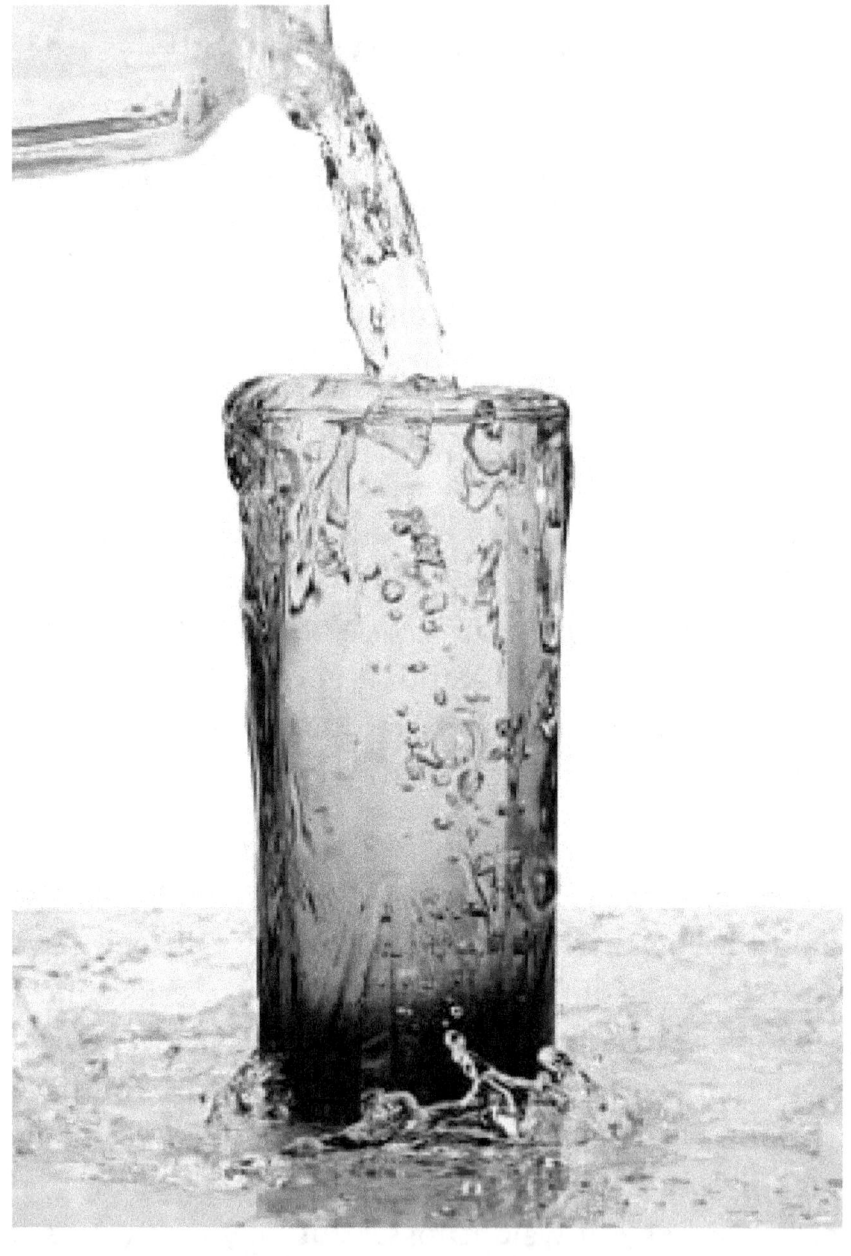

Think of your day, your 24 hours, as a glass. Everything that makes you YOU is the water that fills the glass. Everything. Your job, the friends you spend time with, your hobbies, your family responsibilities, the TV shows you watch, every thought, every emotion. Your life – the glass – is completely full. Now, you decide that you need to lose weight and work out, so, what do you do? You attempt to squeeze dieting and exercising into an already full life. To put it in the context of our glass analogy, you attempt to put more water into an already full glass! This makes the glass of your life overflow, and you quickly find yourself overwhelmed. This is exactly why the marketer in the business of selling weight loss, knows that he can sell an easy, fifteen-minutes-a-day solution to you – it fits into your current life and schedule with no effort. The only catch? **IT DOESN'T WORK**. There is only one way to add fresh water to a full glass, and that is to pour off most of the water already filling the glass. You have to get rid of some parts of your life, some of what makes you YOU. In short, you must become a different person.

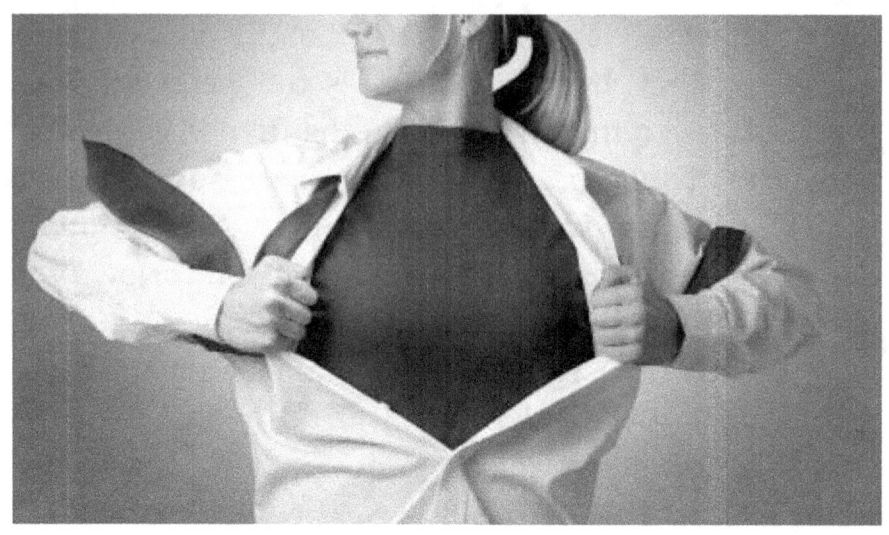

"Lifestyle change" is a phrase that is frequently thrown around to describe the changes necessary to lose weight. Very few people truly understand that phrase in the context of weight loss. Anyone who has lived it knows that becoming a parent, for example, is the ultimate lifestyle change! Even if you are smart enough to realize that becoming a parent is not all bliss and happiness, you can't possibly grasp the impact until the nurse brings your first born to you in your hospital room and neglects to provide the extra 8 hours a day you will need to care for your pride and joy. The lifestyle changes required when you choose to raise a child, absolutely changes you into someone else. That someone else even has a new name: Mom. A mom simply does not live her life as she did when she was childless, or she would be no more than an incubator. It follows that a fit person simply does not live her life as YOU do, or you would be thin.

I recall a discussion with a friend regarding exercise. She admired my dedication to it, and recognized that she needed to exercise regularly, but, "The problem with exercise is that it takes so long to see any difference." I didn't even know how to respond. Suppose you could achieve the body you wanted with only 3 weeks of hard, dedicated exercise. What then? Would you fall back onto the sofa with your chips and remote? Would you fall back into your "normal life?" Wouldn't that be stupid? Wouldn't you soon be right back where you started with 3 weeks wasted? What you need is a NEW normal. No one sets a goal to exercise for a week or even a month. You may not last much longer than that, but your initial goal is to make exercise a part of your regular routine, your lifestyle. If the goal is a lifetime of fitness – 20, 30, or 50 years – why would it matter if it took 6 months or even 6 years to "see any difference?"

Let's say that I decided I wanted to be an airline pilot. This is not likely as I can get lost on the way to the store, much less while crossing the country, but stick with me on this. I would have to give up the gym and the work I do there, make myself available for studying and training, log countless hours at the controls of a plane, and probably have to move to another city. All this before I would be allowed in the cockpit of a plane. If all I wanted was to be a passenger on a flight, hell, I could do that anytime! Most fat people try to achieve a thin life without changing the fat life they currently have. They want a lifetime of fitness in 3 weeks, or the job of airline pilot with the ease of a passenger. You cannot be a part-time fit person, any more than you can be a part-time fat person.

The realization of what it will take to lose weight and keep it off has only just begun to glimmer in your mind. It is an enormous undertaking, one that goes far beyond diet and exercise. Many times along the way you will be tempted to quit – maybe even before you turn the page! Quitting means one of two things: either you are OK with your fat life, or you are delaying the inevitable, because you WILL try to lose weight again.

I've stolen a quote from our website, which I think sums it up nicely... YOU can't lose weight, YOU have tried and YOU have failed. In fact, YOU are incapable of ever losing weight. The real fact is that the only way YOU will lose weight is to stop being YOU!

I welcome your feedback, questions, comments, and experiences. Please share at Donna@StopBeingFat101.com.

2

Stop Being Fat!

Acknowledgement is the first step!

Yes, I'll admit it – I've been accused of being a bit... direct, shall we say. Even harsh. It seems the word "fat" makes people cringe. I'm told there are many gentler synonyms I could be using: overweight, plus-sized, chubby, large, and dozens of others. A well-known personality recently commented on this subject... This is a young lady, the daughter in a famous family, who has recently lost quite a bit of weight and is looking quite fit and healthy these days. She has been through drug rehab to fight a serious addiction problem and is well-known for her foul-mouth, dropping F-bombs like confetti falling at midnight on New Year's Eve. On a recent daytime talk show, she put on her best indignant attitude, and announced that she was offended by the word "fat". Or, maybe it was she was offended by the bleep-ity bleep word "fat", I don't recall exactly. REALLY??? It seems to me that she would be the first to argue that words are nothing more than a combination of letters that describe an idea or object. When did fat become a dirty word?

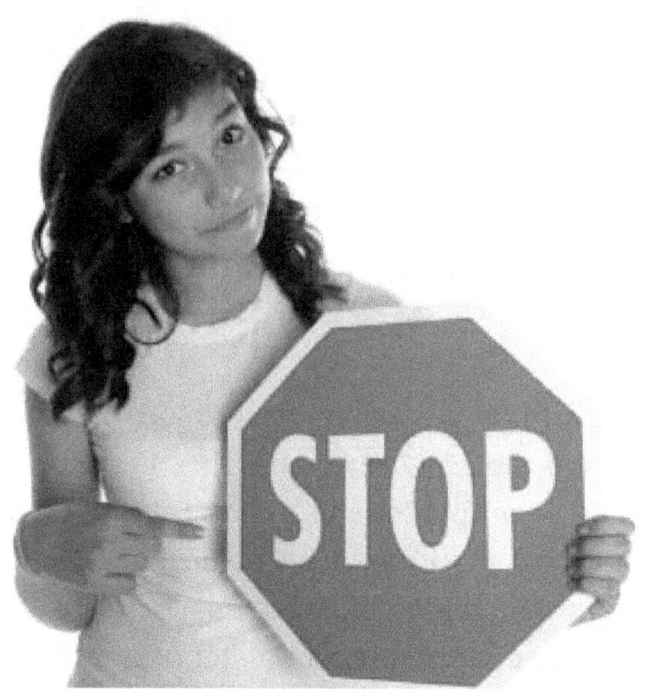

Let's dissect the word overweight, one of the more popular synonyms. The dictionary.com definition of overweight is "weighing too much or more than is considered normal, proper, etc." Luggage can be overweight. Truckloads can be overweight. Does that make either of them fat? For that matter, a 5'8" 275 pound body builder with 5% body fat is certainly overweight. He is definitely NOT fat!

As a noun, thefreedictionary.com defines fat as "adipose tissue, forming soft pads between organs, smoothing and rounding out body contours, and furnishing a reserve supply of energy." As an adjective to describe an individual, we can therefore define fat as "having too much adipose tissue." Is this not exactly what it is? If you've ever gone on a diet or even thought about losing a few pounds, what is it you are trying to lose? Is it hair?...toenails?...muscle? No, it's FAT! I've said it before and truly believe it... if an individual is fat, and completely content and happy with herself, it does NOT bother or concern me in the least. It has **nothing to do with me.** Using the word fat is not about judging or criticizing, it is about the plain, simple truth.

I was a fat kid, from as far back as I can remember. I've heard that vivid memories are often associated with strong emotions. My earliest memory is of my embarrassment at being fat. I was **three and a half years old.** The feeling of embarrassment and humiliation is so clear that I can put those words to that emotion even though I was far too young to know the meaning of either word. Mind you, the people associated with this memory – very dear to me to this day – were not teasing or taunting me, and they never even used the word fat. In fact, I'm 100% CERTAIN if I told them about this painful memory, they would be stunned to know they were responsible. I was not hurt by words or attitudes. I was hurt by my own fatness.

As I became older and started school, I was often teased about being fat by my classmates. Occasionally, a well-meaning adult would intervene. I remember more than one mother telling her daughter or son that I was not fat, I was "pleasantly plump." How I hated that euphemism. Aside from the fact that the term felt demeaning and patronizing, there was not a single thing that was "pleasant" about it. And, the discussion simply prolonged the time when everyone's attention was focused on my weight.

Recently, in our Stop Being Fat Network meeting, we played the "Driver's License Game." I collected everyone's driver's license. Then one by one, I announced the weight on the license and challenged everyone to guess whose license it was. They all sat silent, too polite to speak up. By the end of the game, everyone was laughing at their own self-delusion. Not a single license had the correct weight on it - NOT one. In every case, the weight on the license was off by anywhere from 35 to 75 lbs. One woman reasoned that when she went to bars and was carded, people were actually LOOKING at her license - it was too embarrassing to admit the real weight for the bouncer to read! But, it wasn't too embarrassing to actually BE that weight?? Hmmmm...

When I was a kid, I hardly ever heard the word obese, mainly because one simply did not see that many obese individuals. In the 60s, being described as obese was hurtful and humiliating. Nowadays, we hear the term obesity used daily. Not only has "obesity" become commonplace, the medical community has been forced to roll out a number of new terms to describe our ever "growing" population: morbidly obese, super obese, super-super obese and one I heard recently to describe the worldwide obesity crisis – globesity.

Our society has turned poor choice and an unhealthy lifestyle into the **condition** of obesity.   With the exception of a very, very small percentage of the population, being fat is a personal choice. It's about taking in more calories than your body requires and storing that excess energy as fat. The word fat is not about criticism or judgement, it is about personal responsibility and personal accountability. Stop Being Fat! Yes, it's a choice!

I welcome your feedback, questions, comments, and experiences. Please share at
Donna@StopBeingFat101.com.

3

The Math of Weight Loss

You learned all you need to know about losing weight when you passed your first grade math class!

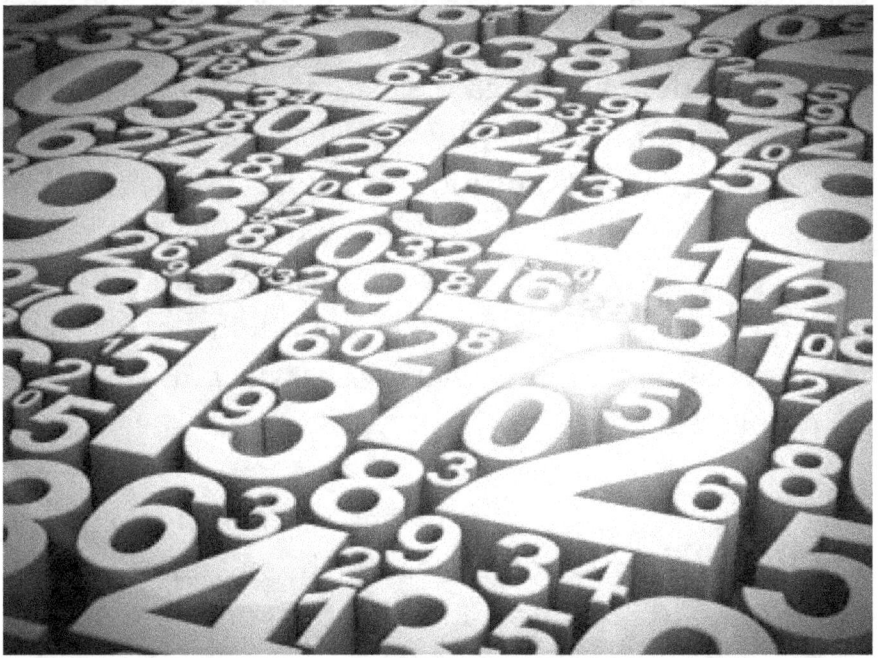

With so many commercials, infomercials and newspaper ads claiming to provide guaranteed weight loss success, it's understandable why people are so confused. Is there really any method, diet or program that works for everyone?

The short answer is NO. Of the thousands of diet books available – be it low-carb, low-fat, or the "toenail diet" (I made that one up there so don't go searching for it) – there will always be someone who follows it and is wildly successful at losing weight while on it. Unfortunately, the vast majority of individuals are sadly unsuccessful. This is not a failing of the diet – they all work if you follow them. As individuals it is not at all important to find a diet that "works for you." It is vitally important, however, to find a diet that you can work with! This would be a balanced diet that provides fewer calories than you burn, and does not contain foods that you cannot stomach, are allergic to, or are problematic for your specific health conditions and/or specialized nutritional needs. There is no "best" diet – the key is the calorie intake. This statement is frustrating to fat individuals who are still looking for the "magic formula for weight loss." Here is a strange, but simple, analogy that may just inspire a light bulb moment.

You stack your sink with dishes after a dinner party. The next day you need a clean dish, so you reach into the cupboard and get another one out rather than wash those already in the sink. You continue this practice until there are no more clean dishes in the house. You now have a choice to make: buy more dishes and just keep adding to the stack, or set about clearing out the sink.

Despite the confusion you may experience when you begin exploring the weight loss section of your local bookstore, losing weight is actually as simple as this analogy suggests. It's a straightforward, daily, add or subtract scenario. Every day, you can put in the effort to rid yourself of the dirty dishes, or you can let those dishes -- weight -- continue to stack up. It's not that people don't get it. People are not stupid. Experience has lead me to believe that fat people are actually OK with being overweight about 80 - 90% of the time. The other 10-20% of the time is spent making the weight loss industry richer. The reverse is true when it comes to fit people. Over indulging on vacations and holidays is OK for a fit person a small percentage of the time. But, they soon become disappointed with themselves and return to their healthy ways. Let me explain what I mean with another analogy.

I would like to have a great singing voice. Imagine standing on a stage in front of 125,000 screaming fans as you belt out Billboard's top selling single. The people who achieve this didn't just wake up one morning with 'Become Superstar' on their 'To Do' list for the day. In most cases, they started with some raw talent and added many years of training and sacrifice. I, on the other hand have zero talent in the singing department, and my desire to reach musical stardom is non-existent. I would, however, like to wake up one morning and be a rock star. That I am **NOT** the next Elvis does not concern me, nor is it on my list of things I need to accomplish. But, if I were handed the keys to Graceland, then, sure, I would take them! I want the rock star life, but my desire is not strong enough to put in the work to achieve it.

Here we can draw a direct parallel, because to want to lose weight and to desire to lose weight are completely different things. In this case, **want** means 'give me' and **desire** means 'work for'. People with the desire to lose weight understand that even if they fill the kitchen sink with 75 sets of dirty dishes, as long as they wash one more than they use every day, eventually there will be no more dirty dishes. People who always have twenty or more pounds of extra weight, want to lose those pounds on any given day, but only desire to lose them when vacations loom or special events beckon. This is why the majority of overweight people will remain fat.

Losing weight and maintaining a weight loss requires a complete lifestyle change, and the truth is most people are not prepared to do that. Instead, they waste their time and money on quick fix, no hope solutions when the mood hits them. This is the 10–20% I was talking about. Don't take my word for it. Just take a close look at yourself and do the math. The secret the weight loss industry doesn't want you to know is that weight loss requires no special diet or any particular exercise equipment –– just figure it out for yourself. If you put more cash in the bank than you take out each month, your balance increases. If you fill your car with gas and don't use it, your car stays full of gas. It really is just a simple equation that anyone can understand, but the businessmen who are committed to parting you from your hard earned cash have done an excellent job convincing people that the way to a slimmer body is through a drink, a pill, or potentially life-threatening surgery.

Many overweight people are, dare I say....Desperate? I am not talking about a few vanity pounds to drop so they can look better on the beach. These people are fat: they look fat, feel fat and consequently are downright miserable. Desperation is the main ingredient in the recipe put together by the multi-billion dollar weight loss industry. People will try anything to lose weight even though every ounce of common sense tells them it's not going to work. They just tell themselves, 'well, worst case scenario, I'll lose some cash.' The very same advertising strategy is aimed at the desperate man who thinks his 'performance' is below par, and figures he has nothing to lose when he opens his wallet for the male enhancement con artists.

If you want to LIVE as a fit person, you have to BECOME that fit person -- and not just 20% of the time. That, in a nutshell, is the Stop Being Fat philosophy. It's not about promoting a special diet or tricking you into a program with 'lose all the weight you want for 5 dollars a week' -- oh, and did we mention that supplements are part of the deal and they cost a lot more? Stop

Being Fat is the simple, honest philosophy of teaching you the habits of a fit person. Those habits are then reinforced with a fabulous payoff -- losing weight! I want to help you drop that first 5 pounds in way that you can carry forward to drop the next 20 or next 100, AND keep it off. If you are ready to do the work, if you are ready to become that fit person, **Stop Being Fat** is ready to show you how -- analogies included!

I welcome your feedback, questions, comments, and experiences. Please share at Donna@StopBeingFat101.com.

4

Quit Looking for the Shortcut

Why are otherwise reasonable people certain that "fast and easy" weight loss is possible, even when they've never been able to find it?

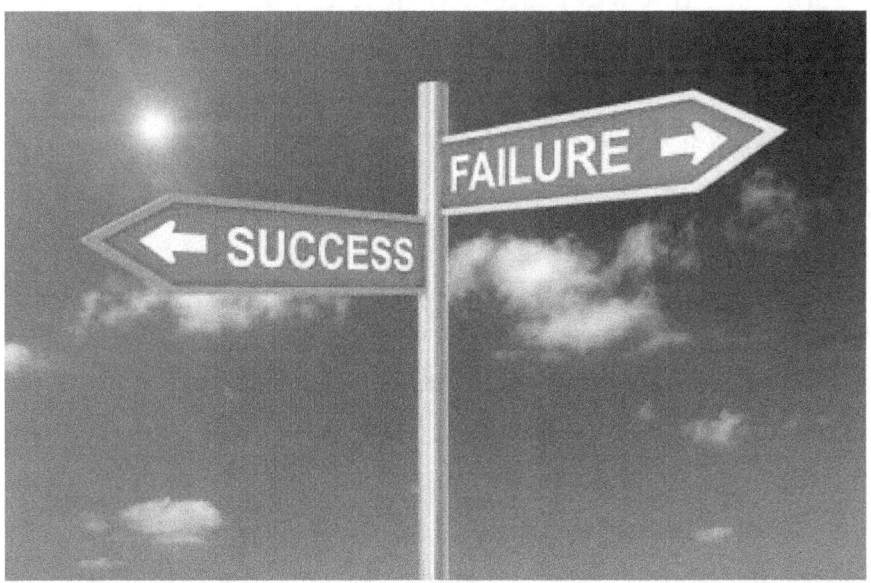

A friend of mine launching a new online workout, recently took an internet course through a local university. One of the topics covered in the course was search engine optimization (SEO) – techniques used by the technically savvy to return your website at the top of the list when a keyword search is performed. Through an exercise designed to illustrate the importance of SEO, she learned an interesting tidbit of information: there are easily one million searches

every day for "weight loss", "fat loss", "weight control" and other variations of that theme.

A million searches a day? Really???

Why then aren't weight loss programs filled to capacity? Why aren't gyms turning people away and making money hand over fist? The answer is simple: people are not interested in how to lose weight. They are interested in how to lose weight **easily.** If you are one of those people looking for easy weight loss, you may as well look for a unicorn – you'd have a better chance of finding it.

Our drive–thru, fast food, labor saving, instant gratification, make–life–more–convenient society has contributed to our epidemic of obesity. It now threatens the solution – we are not interested in the hard work and commitment required to achieve and maintain a healthy lifestyle. I, myself, am guilty of the expectation of convenience. When I plan a trip, my first step is always to look for an airline to take me there. Not only would I rather fly than drive, but I expect the flight to be completely affordable, and I complain if the airline does not see fit to transport me non–stop! My expectation of convenience doesn't end with my vacation, either. More often than I care to admit, mealtime involves a can opener, microwave, automatic dishwasher and occasionally – when even those three appliances are too demanding – the phone number of my favorite carryout restaurant.

Think about the last time a friend, relative or co-worker gave you the news about her pregnancy. Did you ask, "So, how long do you plan to grow the baby?" Of course not. It takes nine months. Did your friend ask you to suggest a doctor who would produce the expected baby a few months earlier because spring was going to be a more convenient time of year than summer? Of course not. It takes nine months. While some parents would argue that nine months isn't anywhere NEAR enough time to prepare for the trauma...uh, joy of parenthood, the idea of a shortcut isn't even part of the discussion.

Recently, I posted my own weight loss success story on a blogging site along with a photo. I received a great deal of feedback, but there were two questions in particular that I found very interesting....

One woman explained how she had already lost 18 pounds, but it was coming off too slowly for her, about a pound a week. She was at 1500 calories a day, and could not cut any more from her diet. Nor could she add any more exercise – after all, a person needed a little down time to relax after a full day at work. Her question to me was, "How can I jump start my weight loss?" My simple answer, "You can't." She was doing exactly what was required for her to lose one pound a week. To expect to lose 2 or 3 pounds a week without changing anything she was doing was unreasonable.

Another woman congratulated me on my amazing loss and fit body. Her question was, "What's your secret?" The secret is there is no secret. Despite the fact that my blog explained the months of hard work and exercise it had taken, she was certain there was a still more – a secret she was not privy to!

You know where this is going so I won't state the obvious. But, let me plant a seed... This time next year is going to come around whether you want it to or not. This time next year, you can still be out-of-shape, overweight, and using Google® to find the magic pill for weight loss. Or, you can be 20, 50, 100 pounds lighter. Think about it.

I welcome your feedback, questions, comments, and experiences. Please share at
Donna@StopBeingFat101.com.

5

Results Not Typical

Stop believing the "fast and easy weight loss" con men.

Lose weight in 5 minutes a day!
Eat what you want and lose weight!
Shed unwanted pounds without working out!
Burn fat as you sleep!

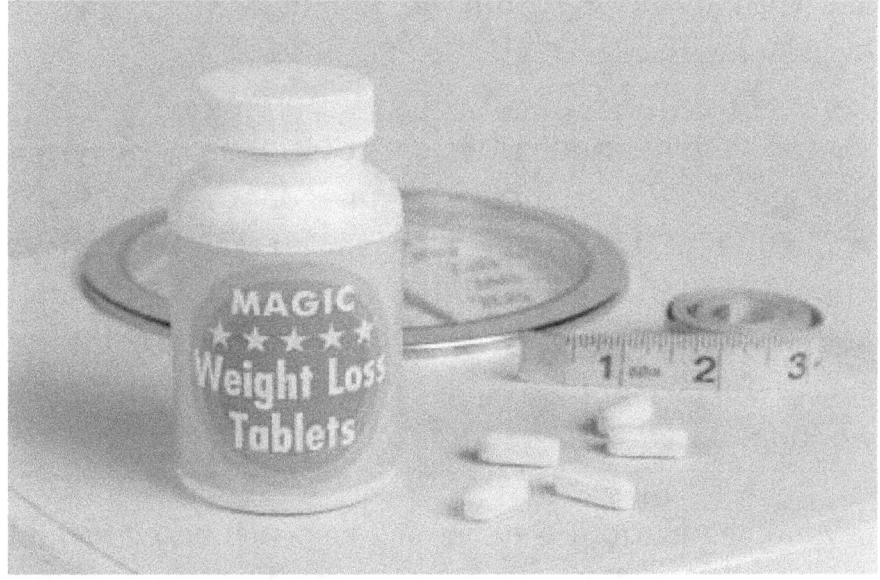

You've seen the ads on TV, in magazines and on billboards: lean, fit, men and bikini clad women flashing bright smiles and six pack abs, all achieved through use of the latest, greatest weight loss product! You are eager to believe, eager to part with your hard earned cash in the hope that maybe, just maybe, science has finally uncovered the effortless formula for magical weight loss. But, wait...squint a little and take a closer look at the fine print....

These claims have not been substantiated.
When combined with diet and regular exercise.
Results not typical.

Crank up your healthy skepticism and think about it for one minute. If there **was** a pill that could deliver weight loss with a glass of water and your daily vitamin, you wouldn't be reading about it in an advertisement. **It would be the lead story on the nightly news.**

The multi-billion dollar weight loss industry does not run on fact or science. It runs on the successful marketing of the simple concept of eat less, move more. Year after year, studies tell us that – no matter how it is packaged – the bottom line when it comes to successful weight loss is restricting calories and working out. Period.

Several years ago, I watched a TV special about weight loss. The producers had assembled a panel of ten dietary "experts" and assigned to them the task of selecting THE best diet for losing weight. Each diet presented had elements that the panel, as a whole, could agree were beneficial. But, none of them – for various reasons – could possibly be everything to everybody. As individuals, we all have different nutritional requirements based on our medical history, age, gender, and a host of other reasons. Each panel member stubbornly adhered to their personal recommendation. Not surprisingly, they all had a book to sell! In the end, the ONLY consensus they could reach was that a good diet needed to be balanced, and would always work if the dieter took in fewer calories than they burned. End of story. Not even a Super Bowl® ad, however, could effectively sell "cut your calories, workout daily, be uncomfortable, lose weight." How do you separate the BS from the truth?

When you read or hear an ad, take it at face value – never assume that a statement **implies** anything. A friend of mine – Sue – returned from lunch at work one day with a fitness magazine she had purchased. The cover blared "Get Six Pack Abs Without Difficult Crunches!" A quick glance at the article, and I broke the bad news: true enough, crunches were NOT part of this abs routine, but every exercise recommended was, in fact, more difficult than a standard crunch. A more honest cover would have said "Six Pack Abs in 3 Easy Lessons....and 10 Extremely Difficult Ones!", but, of course, THAT would not have enticed Sue to buy the magazine.

When it comes to pills and supplements, read the directions carefully and completely, and mentally translate it to what that means in your daily routine. I had a recent discussion with a friend who had bought into an expensive supplement that was supposed to boost her metabolism, thereby accelerating weight loss. It seems she had to take the supplement 4 times a day, with 2 glasses of water, no closer than 2 hours within any meal (before or after). In addition, there were restrictions on how soon she could eat her first meal of the day and how late she could eat her last. It didn't take a math genius to realize that in a 16 hour day, there were SOOO many hours where she was not allowed to eat, she was – by default – cutting her calories. She wasn't doing anything unhealthy. Cutting calories and drinking loads of water are important elements in any weight loss program. But, she WAS paying someone else a great deal of money for what?...her own self discipline and a tablet full of useless herbs.

Beware of guarantees, in particular, the "up to" escape clause. "Lose up to 20 pounds and more in 5 weeks or your money back!" "Increases your metabolism up to 200% within the first week or return the product for a full refund!" The fact that 0 is always on the way when you count "up to" 20, 200, anything really, ensures that retailers will never return a cent to disillusioned consumers.

No doubt you are thinking that surely SOME of the weight loss products you've seen advertised must be effective. The ads frequently include testimonials from success stories or doctors who present scientific evidence of the product effectiveness – or is it just a guy in a white coat that you assumed is a doctor? Still not convinced? Consider this: professional boxers – those who are featured on Pay Per View® channels and are often the center of much media hype – are among the fittest of athletes. One bout can be worth millions to a pro boxer. And, while a boxer gets a huge check, win or lose, he MUST tip the scale in his weight class in order to fight the bout and earn his payoff. In short, the number on the scale is worth MILLIONS to him. So, what does he do? He runs, he jumps rope, he hits the bag until his shoulders feel like jelly. He sweats and swears and works his ass off. If a six-minute-a-day workout or a bottle of "metabo-bollocks" would allow a boxer to reach his weight goal, he would use it!!!

There are as many ways to market weight loss products as there are desperate people willing to take a chance on them. The best way to protect yourself from the scam artists?...accept that the only REAL way to lose weight, become fit, and stay that way is to embrace the lifestyle changes necessary: eat less, move more. It works every time. Results ARE typical!

I welcome your feedback, questions, comments, and experiences. Please share at
Donna@StopBeingFat101.com.

6

I Knew that Damn Shower Curtain Was Making Me Fat!

And other tall tales to tell around the camp fire!

There is a massive interest in weight loss – that it is a multi-billion dollar industry bears this out. As such, weight loss is never out of the news, the talk shows or reality TV. It is BIG business and competition for advertising dollars is fierce and relentless!

As such, the media is constantly searching for new information when it comes to, weight loss and everything related to it.Every talk show, every news program, every magazine wants to reel us in. Grabbing our attention translates directly to advertising dollars. Think about the daytime talk shows. Year after year we see segments that promise to deliver the "miracle food" that is essential to weight loss, the "number one" exercise for fat loss, or the "hidden danger" that is making you fat.

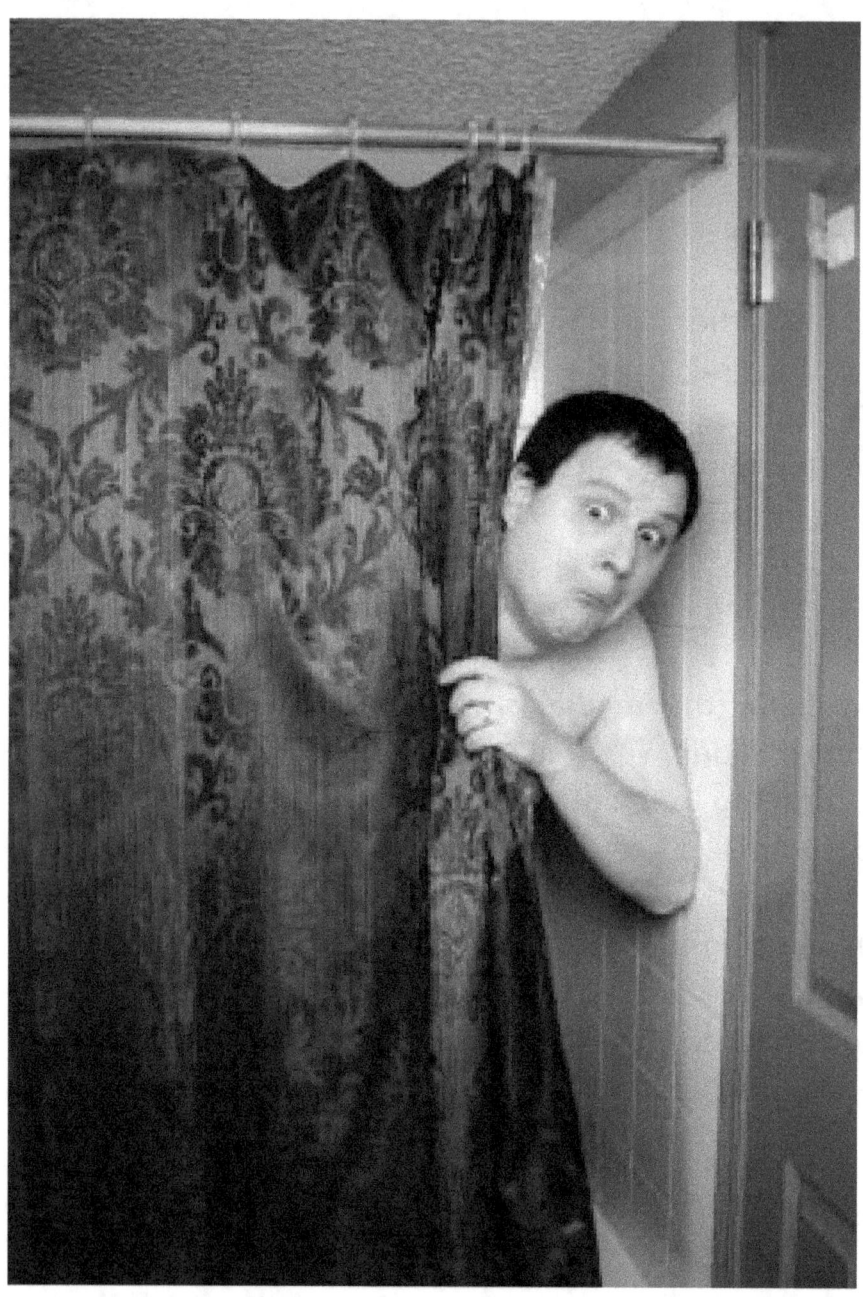

I've learned that not enough sleep can make me fat –
as a single mother working two jobs, it's amazing I
don't weigh 300 pounds as I have not had a full night's

rest since 1988. Did you know, too, that walnuts have omega-3 fatty acids which can help burn fat. A side of walnuts with your burger and fries is just what the doctor ordered! And, listen to this one...sitting in a bath of ice is sure to help you lose weight! As long as we eat our pizza in the bathroom, no harm done, right? I've heard every one of these "revelations" on daytime TV.

Remember the "fat gene" discovered a few years ago and the subject of many newspaper headlines and news show stories? British scientists had uncovered a gene that was common to many obese people, leading them to conclude there was a gene that contributed to obesity. Many fat people jumped on the fat gene theory – it was a ready made excuse for their obesity. The only problem with this excuse was that genetic tendencies within a population generally develop over thousands or even hundreds of thousands of years – it's called evolution. Obesity is a relatively recent problem, only within the last 50-75 years at most. Is it more likely that Mother Nature burdened two thirds of the American population with a fat gene in the last 50 years, or that our population has become fatter and fatter due to a more sedentary lifestyle, and a prevalence of labor saving devices and convenience foods?

And, then there were "obesogens", chemicals found in plastics, pesticides and other non-natural substances which contribute to obesity. According to daytime TV, obesogens are prevalent in our food supply and present in many plastics we come in contact with on a daily basis – everything from the plastic containers where we store our leftovers to our plastic shower curtains. Again, fat people jumped on the obesogen bandwagon. It is far easier to blame the environment than to take responsibility for being fat. With obesogens attacking our waistlines continually, how is it possible that ANYONE is thin? Do thin people never take showers? Do they shop at different stores than fat people do?

And, how many times have you tuned into your favorite daytime TV show where the scheduled guest has a fantastic new plan guaranteed to be the last diet you will ever need – detailed, of course, in his new book which has conveniently JUST hit the bookstores at $24.95! These days, daytime TV looks a lot more like an hour long infomercial than it does an hour of entertainment.

Of course, there is the tiniest shred of truth in everything mentioned above. The problem is that each is but one piece in a 1000-piece jigsaw puzzle and 950 of the pieces are diet and exercise. The danger comes from the sensational presentation by the media, which offers up these stories as if they alone are reporting the breaking news that explains it all! Fat people are far too willing to accept any answer that provides an easy solution or any excuse that deflects the blame away from them and outside their control. The easy way out will always be preferred. Eat less, move more will never be the basis of a daily show!

I'm not asking you to give up your news, your talk shows or your reality TV. They can be highly entertaining and informative. I'm only asking that when it comes to weight loss, understand that what you are seeing and hearing is the result of marketing strategy not scientific discovery. When all is said and done and yesterday's premiere episode of the new season is today's rerun, the simple concept of calories in, calories out is the only weight loss truth that you can't shoot holes through.

I welcome your feedback, questions, comments, and experiences. Please share at
Donna@StopBeingFat101.com.

7

Don't Kid Yourself

Fat individuals are masters at denial.

Being overweight can affect your health, your energy and your self esteem. Almost everyone knows this, even individuals who have never been fat. What most people don't realize – fat or otherwise – is how fat people kid themselves on a regular, even daily basis. Kid themselves? What does THAT mean?

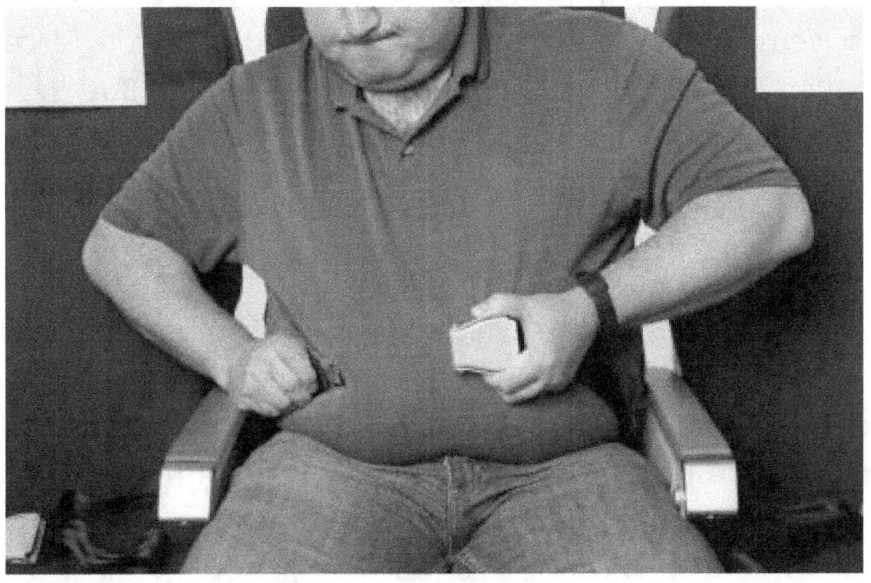

One of the tools used in our weight loss program at the gym is a weight loss game. This game is designed to motivate individuals to lose weight thru a series of colorful bracelets. The constant visual measure of a participant's progress (or lack thereof!) is a

TREMENDOUS accountability tool! As such, one of the rules of the game is that it must be played 24/7, and participants who show up without their bracelets are taken to task. One such "cheater" admitted that she had removed the bracelet because she went to a black tie event and it "didn't look good with my diamond tennis bracelet." **And, her oversized behind did?** She laughed at that blunt statement, but could not deny it. Don't kid yourself.

Another common form of denial I see are those program participants who do not want their weight posted for tracking their progress. Weight, of course, is sensitive personal information and I don't force anyone to publicly announce their weight. But, lets face it – I don't need to know the number on the scale to know that an individual is fat. Don't kid yourself.

Denial has a serious side, too. The list of health risks associated with obesity is extensive: everything from type 2 diabetes, heart disease, sleep apnea, some cancers, and on and on it goes. You can't imagine the number of fat individuals I've met who are not worried about their type 2 diabetes. They have their diabetes under control with medication. Think again. Diabetes can be **managed** with medication, not controlled. Don't kid yourself.

What type of vacations do fat people take? Warm, sunny locations involving bathing suits and beaches are out of the question, as are hiking trips or sightseeing activities involving a lot of walking. Some folks don't even venture beyond a destination where they would be required to squeeze into an airline seat! Don't kid yourself. And, airplanes are not the only place where the seats are unforgiving. What about movies, concerts, sporting events or the theater? Don't kid yourself.

Everyone has bad days when they are trying to diet – many people have them regularly. There will always, ALWAYS be an excuse to party – a birthday, reunion, wedding, whatever. Those who don't seem to be able to get thru a week without cheating frequently defend themselves with "Well, you gotta live!" Hauling around 50, 60, 100 or more extra pounds ... how is THAT living? Sore back, stressed joints, expensive medications. Don't kid yourself.

In the Stop Being Fat weight loss program at my gym, it is easy to spot a fat person who has figured out what is required to lose weight and who is doing everything right. Oddly enough, identifying that person has little to do with the pounds that are coming off.
They are energetic, enthused, and confident. Conversely, it is easy to spot a fat person who has lost that "mojo" or who still hasn't found it. And, we are not afraid to call them on it by pointing out that if they are not living by "What Would a Thin Person Do?" they are certain to be heavier this time next year. One

hundred percent of the time, the reply is, "No way am I going to put the weight back on." Really? If you are not doing what is required to lose weight, gain is inevitable. You will NOT stay the same. Think about it. If, living your current life, you could have stopped gaining weight, why didn't you do it 20, 50, 100 pounds ago? I am the Master of Weight Maintenance. My weight is always going **up** or going **down.** I don't just sit at 112 lbs. week in and week out. Don't kid yourself.

If you are fat, you've probably seen yourself in one of the examples cited above. Some serious thought will likely reveal some other areas of your life where your weight is controlling, affecting or denying you the life you deserve. Take back control. Do it now.

I welcome your feedback, questions, comments, and experiences. Please share at Donna@StopBeingFat101.com.

8

You Are Not the Exception

As much as you would like to be off the hook for not losing weight, you do not get excused!

One of the programs offered at my gym is a weight loss motivation and exercise education program designed to enable participants to lose 20 pounds in 10 weeks. With each session, the results vary from wildly successful to mediocre. But, while the results can never be predicted, I can always count on one thing: There is at least person who, whether she knows it or not, is really not there to lose weight. She is there to be "excused."

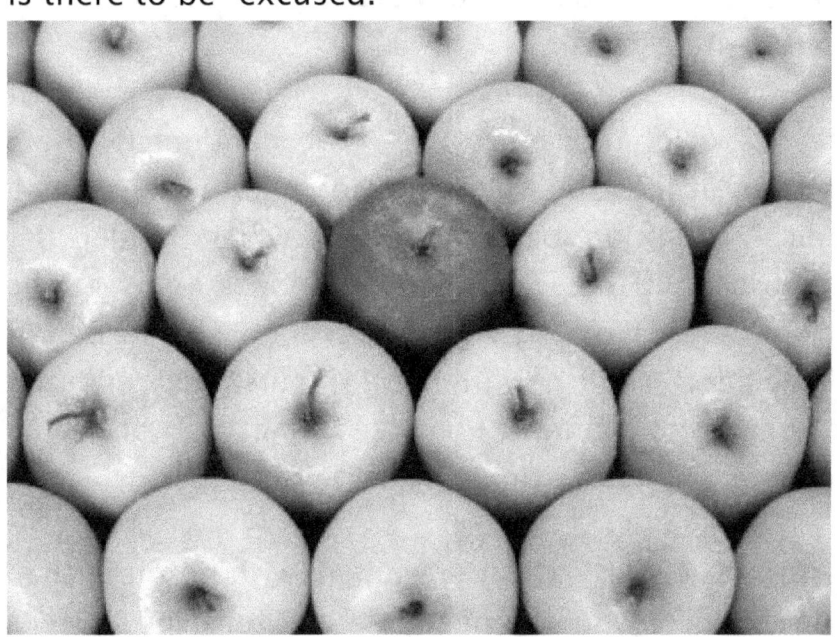

Typically, this person has tried and failed to lose weight for years. Diets "don't work" for her. She is too busy, her metabolism is too slow, NO ONE could possibly have more to deal with in their life than she does. She is there because she wants to hear, "By golly, you are right! Your life is simply too busy, your responsibilities too great. You are not to blame for your obesity." For every solution you offer her to overcome a challenge she faces, she has a reason for why that won't work. She is "the exception."

"I can't trust my husband to take care of the kids." "My friends give me grief when I don't drink and eat." "My hairstyle takes an hour every night." (Yikes!) Believe it or not, every one of the above excuses has been used by participants in our program. My personal favorite: "I have a lot of plants to water." (Are the plants in different states??!)

In every weight loss session we've conducted, there has been at least one person who is certain she has a medical condition or "tendencies" which hinder her weight loss. If the scale does not show a loss, yet she tells me she is eating right, I have no choice but to believe her. I can't be with her 24 hours a day. I'm not the one who suffers if indeed she is not being completely honest with me or herself.

I recall one client – a young woman, with no more than 20 lbs to lose, who had been 'dieting' for over 4 weeks and had not lost a pound. She was, by her account, eating no more than 700 calories a day – far too little. Additionally, I saw her work out on a regular basis and knew she worked out HARD.   If her calorie count was accurate, she wasn't eating enough to support her 1 hour workout, much less her entire day. She insisted there must be "something wrong" with her metabolism. I had a suspicion she was not being entirely truthful about her diet, so before suggesting she see a doctor, I asked her to record everything she ate for a week. I know a couple of people who write down everything they eat every day and have for years. Most people can't and don't need to spend their lifetime monitoring every morsel they eat.   But, it can be a very useful exercise for a week or two. Often times you discover a lot of "careless calories" you did not realize you were taking in. We often dip into the candy jar or grab from the chip bowl purely out of habit. The simple process of recording what you eat makes you more careful, especially if you think someone else is going to be scrutinizing your journal!

But, back to our young friend... When the week passed and she showed me her food journal, it was clear that she had no concept of calorie counting. Admittedly, she had been guessing about the calories in many foods she was eating – 10 chicken hot wings, for example, were counted as 50 calories! ("Well, there isn't hardly any meat on them.") The seven hundred calories she had carefully counted for purposes of proving to me that she was simply not able to lose weight as easily as everyone else, turned out to be about 1200 calories. And, NOT coincidentally, she managed to lose 4 pounds the week she was logging her calories for me to check! From that point on, her weight loss was easy.

I recall a discussion with another client (call her H2-no) about retraining herself to drink more water – important for successful weight loss. I built this habit for myself by taking a glass of water with me EVERY time I got in my car. The water was right next to me, always ready to be sipped. **BUT**...H2-no never drove far enough to finish off a glass of water. I pointed out that she could accomplish the same thing by keeping a glass of water on her desk at work. **BUT**...the ice in the glass would melt before H2-no could finish the water, and the water HAD to be cold. I suggested that H2-no bring refillable containers of water to work and keep them in the office fridge. She could then use a smaller mug, and keep the ice fresh all day with trips to the freezer, if necessary. **BUT**...and I quote, "Donna, I'm not going to mess with carrying in water or walking to the refrigerator to get more ice!" When it became clear I was not about to declare her the exception and agree that she could not drink all the water she needed, she simply decided I was the unreasonable one!

One of my favorite cartoons shows a doctor counseling a patient. The patient is obese, in his underwear and wearing a startled expression as the doctor asks, "What fits your busy schedule better, exercising one hour a day or being dead 24 hours a day?" In our 24/7, run and race world, finding time to make your fitness and health a priority will be one of the biggest challenges you face. But, no one is a helpless victim of circumstance – the control is in your hands.

I welcome your feedback, questions, comments, and experiences. Please share at Donna@StopBeingFat101.com.

9

Learn to Be Selfish

You are the only one who can make you a top priority.

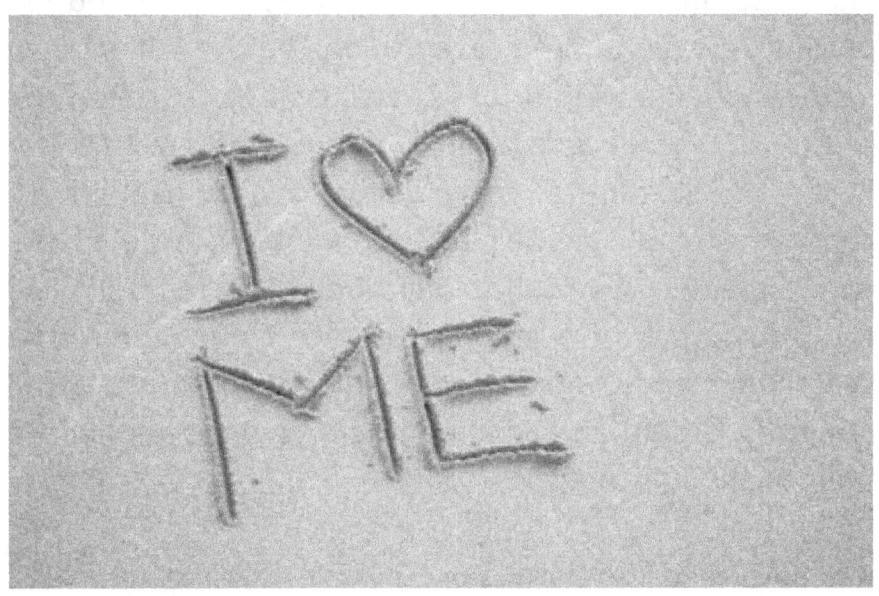

Share. It is drilled into our heads beginning at a very young age – typically the first time we scream "MINE!" and grab our favorite toy from the hands of a playmate. Early on we are encouraged to share treats with our siblings, the ball with our friends, crayons with our classmates. As we grow from toddler to preteen and onward we learn that sharing is not only essential to our social maturity, but actually has a payback – we feel good about sharing! By the time we are adults, with significant others and children of our own, our life is built around sharing, compromising, and putting the needs of others first.

To succeed at weight loss, **you must learn to be selfish**. You need to demand and take what is right for you, and do it with no guilt or apologies.

Mothers, in particular, are spectacularly good at putting everyone and everything before their own needs. When a weight loss client has been missing her workouts, the excuse almost always starts with, "The kids ...." a) started soccer practice, b) needed 50 cupcakes for a school party, c) wanted a ride to the movie theater, or d) all of the above. Take your pick. Every loving mom wants to protect her children and see them happy. Teaching them not to run into the street is essential. Making their favorite dinner on their birthday is not.

I've exercised regularly since I was 11 years old. As a single mom with 2 children, getting my workouts in was often an exercise in logistics, but I rarely missed a scheduled workout. When my daughter became 13, the grumbling started. Why did I have to be away soooo much? Why was the gym sooooo important? I felt guilty – for about a week. I realized that, at age 13, she was building a social life. She was old enough to have a large network of friends, but too young to get in a car and go see them, or to be out on the town with them by herself. In essence, my social butterfly was bored when she was home by herself! When this became clear to me, I said to her, "I've always worked out on this schedule, and it isn't going to change. Find something to do for an hour and a half. I am not the entertainment committee." Incredibly enough, she did not end up in therapy!

When you begin to create the new you – to pour some of your life out of the glass and replace it with elements that support your new healthy lifestyle – you are absolutely affecting everyone around you. Many of those close to you will not be happy. Oh, sure, they are all for it when you start; it sounds like a great idea. Until it affects THEIR life. Until you no longer want to go out and party on Saturdays; or when you replace your awesome homemade fried chicken and mashed potatoes with grilled fish and veggies; or when you can't volunteer at school because you need to be at the gym. You have every right to strive for higher self esteem and a better quality of life for yourself. But, understand the transition will be difficult. YOU are the one making the waves – they were quite happy with life before you decided to get healthy.

No one cares about you. That's a pretty harsh statement. OF COURSE, people care about you! They love you. They want you to be happy. They worry when you are ill or troubled. But, anyone who is "put out" by your attempts to get healthier and feel better about yourself, only resents that you aren't willing to do the things and live the way THEY want you to! They are thinking of themselves and how your self improvement project has had a ripple affect on them. It is not that they don't care – but they don't think about how your decisions affect you, they only think about how it affects them.

I recall a recent discussion with one of our Stop Being Fat Network participants. She signed on for 10 weeks with a goal to lose 20 pounds, and to use that kick start to continue to lose the additional 80 pounds she was carrying. In 10 weeks, she lost 28 pounds. On her last day in the program, she confessed to frustration with her husband. He had been counting the days until the 10 weeks were up. As she headed to her last SBFN meeting, he'd grumbled, "Good, that means this will all be over after today." To her, this 28 pounds was just the start. She was understandably concerned that all her hard work was for nothing, as she didn't expect him to support her continued attempts to drop the rest of the weight. In the end, they reached a compromise. The last time we talked, her weight loss had slowed down considerably – she had agreed not to be all-obsessive in her weight loss and fitness goals. For his part, he agreed to join her with his own self improvement project – to go to the gym with her, and to eat healthy at least PART of the time. She was willing to compromise for him because he was so important to her. But, she was not willing to give up on her dream simply because it wasn't HIS dream.   She learned to be selfish.

As you make the transition from the fat you to the thin you, you may lose some friends along the way.   Do NOT feel guilty or responsible.   It simply means that the new you is not what they signed on for when you became friends.   Being selfish is not always a bad thing. You cannot be truly happy with yourself unless you start with being true to yourself.

I welcome your feedback, questions, comments, and experiences. Please share at Donna@StopBeingFat101.com.

10

Get Over It!
Wallowing in self pity
achieves zip, zero, zilch!

"It's just not fair!"

In my years counseling people on weight loss, I can't tell you how many times I've heard this complaint. Usually, it is spoken by a middle-aged woman who has struggled for weeks to drop a pound, only to see her husband drop 5 pounds in a weekend when he cuts his daily ice cream habit from 3 to 2 scoops. There will always be people that stay thin with no effort. There will always be people who don't understand OR sympathize with your challenge. Mother Nature is an unfair sea hag and there is only one thing you can do about it: **GET OVER IT!**

Before you dismiss me as one of the unsympathetic, I am, in fact, one of those who struggled with weight issues as far back as I can remember. My earliest memories, (3 ½ years old) are associated with my embarrassment at being overweight. To add insult to injury, my 6 brothers and sisters were all skinny! Feeling sorry for myself accomplished nothing. At the age of 19, I was over 200 pounds. Eventually, I figured it out and lost over 85 pounds. I got over it. You need to do the same.

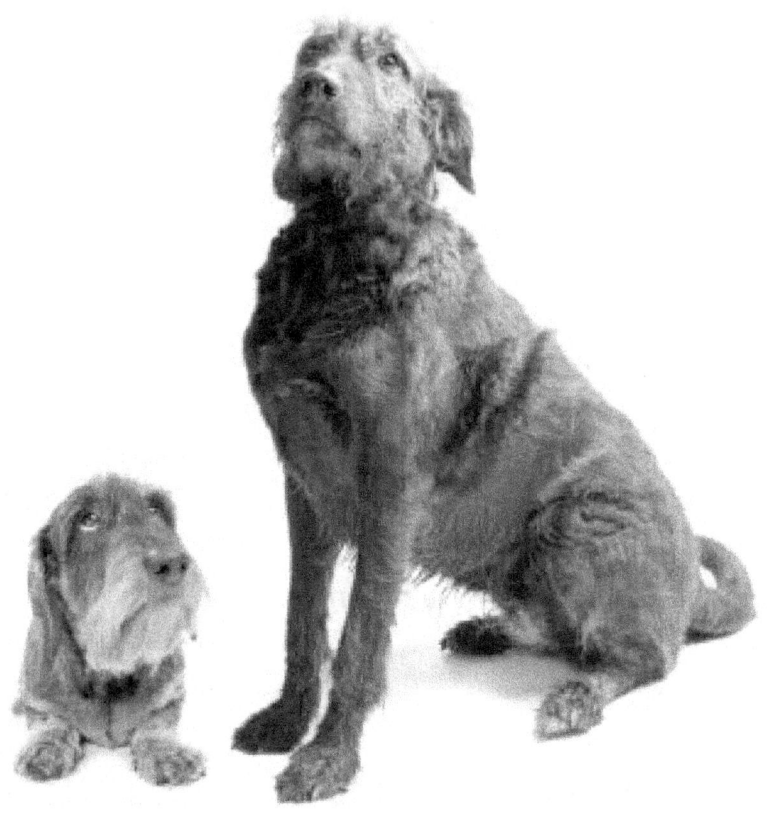

One of my business partners is a 52 yr old man – a former competitive athlete, incredibly fit to this day, and not at all familiar with the difficulties of losing and/or maintaining a healthy weight with a history of weight problems and a slow metabolism. For years I argued with him that he needed to be more sympathetic with fat people, particularly women. All women know that men (generally) lose weight easier – MUCH easier. In all those years of debating, his response never changed – "Not relevant. Doesn't matter." It was frustrating to me that he was so indifferent to my reality, and the reality of many women. One day, in a flash of brilliance, he opened my eyes with the perfect analogy...

I am 5'1" tall. I can't reach the top shelf of my kitchen cupboard – not even on my tip toes. My son is just shy of 6 feet. He can reach anything on the top shelf, AND taunt me with short jokes all at the same time! If he is not in the kitchen, I have to go to the closet, get a stool, and climb the stool to achieve my goal. Genetically, I was "cheated" in the height department and my son was blessed. Does that mean I can't get items off the top shelf of my cupboard? Not at all – it simply means it requires more effort on my part.

So, too, with weight loss. In order to lose weight, it might be necessary for you to workout 6 times a week and cut your intake to 1200 calories a day. For your best friend, 2 workouts a week and 1800 calories might do the trick. This is frustrating, maddening and yes, damn unfair, but **it doesn't change the requirement!** Weight loss has nothing to do with what fits your schedule, what you want to do, or what you have time to do. Yes, you can be stubborn and decide that you are going to do exactly what your friend does to lose weight because – well, that's fair. Stay fat then. Let's face it, if losing weight was easy, we would all be thin and fit.

Mother Nature has cheated and blessed us all in different ways. It's unfortunate that weight loss woes can't be solved with a trip to the closet to get the stool. But, the principle is the same. The reward WILL be worth the effort. It isn't fair. But, it is achievable.

I welcome your feedback, questions, comments, and experiences. Please share at Donna@StopBeingFat101.com.

11

Don't Let the Scale Beat You

Don't fixate on a number, work for a feel.

A recent TV ad for a weight loss product cast an amusing light on a common issue that creates a lot of discussion with our weight loss clients. The ad shows a chubby gentleman stepping on a scale. He steps off the scale and runs around for 10–15 seconds, whereupon he hops back on the scale, his facial expression displaying eager excitement at what he anticipates will surely be a weight loss. Of course, he is disappointed when there is no loss.

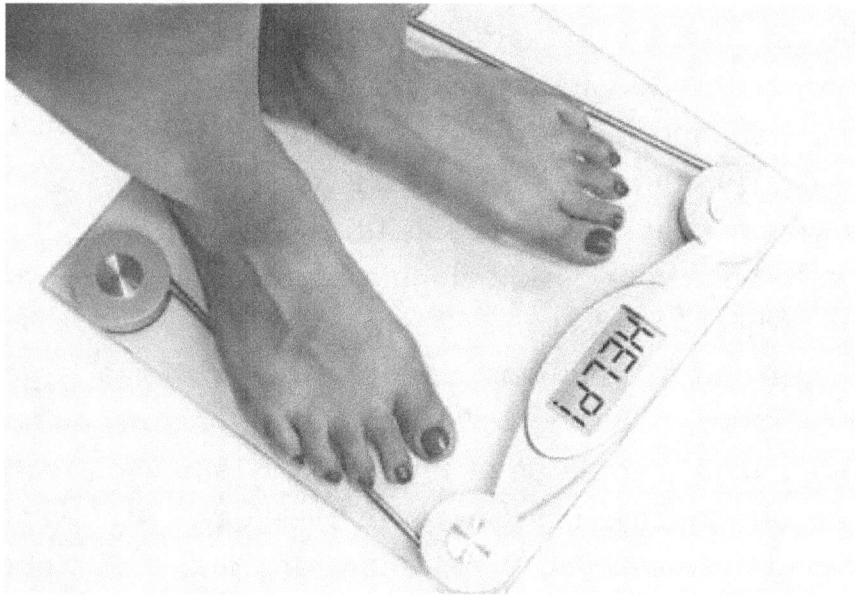

If you have ever tried to lose weight, the scale can be your best friend and your worst enemy. Like our chubby friend above, too many of our clients overuse the scale, often weighing themselves daily or even several times a day. The confidence boost that comes with days of disciplined eating and regular exercise can be undone in the seconds it takes for our digital friend to issue the bad news. I weigh myself once a week, always on the same day at the same time. I'm in maintenance mode, of course, but this was true even when I was in weight loss mode. I knew that no good would come of stepping on the scale too often. A weight gain from one day to the next would depress me and put me into a why-bother-even-trying mode. By contrast, a weight loss would make me over confident and put me into an I-can-ease-up mode. Both were an invitation to fall off the diet wagon.

It's an extreme example, but I recall trying – unsuccessfully – to convince one such "scale addict" that weighing herself a self-admitted EIGHT TIMES A DAY was nothing less that weight loss sabotage. Many of you reading this have full-time jobs which require you to be at your desk, behind a counter, or perhaps at the wheel of a truck each morning at a time determined by your boss. I used to work for a large corporation as a programmer. I knew if I set my alarm for 5:30am, I could be at my desk by 7am. That was true on Monday, Tuesday, every weekday. As I went through my morning preparation for work, it was not necessary to continual check the time on my clock to make sure I could get to work by 7am. Years of the same hair, make-up and dressing routine had taught me that 5:30am was my "snooze you lose" time if I was going to be to work at 7am. Continually checking the clock to see the time was not necessary and in fact, would have likely proven to be counter-productive – it would have made me late!

It sounds contradictory for a weight loss expert to downplay the importance of the scale, but think of it this way: the scale is a tool, a compass, if you will. A compass will never replace a map, it simply tells you that you are headed in the right direction. If you are actively trying to lose fat pounds, you **do** want to see a trend on the scale that says "yes, I am moving closer to Fitville." But, to allow a weight gain now and again to discourage you or – even worse – completely derail your efforts, is a trap that many discouraged dieters fall into and never escape from.

Hundreds of people have come to my gym, seeking help in achieving their weight loss goals. NONE of those people came to me because of a number seen on the scale. They came to me because of what they saw in the mirror. They don't like how their clothes fit or how they feel about themselves. Funny how these very same people will notice some extra room in their clothes, will gain a spring in their step and a smile that reflects their improving self image – only to kamikaze their efforts with a resurgence of self loathing when they see an extra pound one day. I start every weight loss group with the same warning – for purposes of our Stop Being Fat Network, your progress will be gauged by MY scale, at the same time every week. Don't complain to me about what it says. I don't care about your scale at home! Inevitably, every single participant steps on the gym scale at some point, gasps, and exclaims, "MY scale says I am down!" The average bathroom scale costs $20-$50. To expect NASA-like precision from every scale is completely delusional! I can move my own scale from the wood flooring in my kitchen to the tile in my foyer and get a different reading in the same house in the same minute, for heaven's sake!

Weight gain and loss is an emotional issue for many people, so it is difficult to not allow the scale to determine your mood. You want to average a one or two pound loss each week you are trying to lose weight, but the key word is **average.** For women in particular, weight can fluctuate on any given day for reasons that have nothing to do with actual fat loss or gain (hormones, water retention, stress, etc., etc.). It's the consistent dedication to your diet and exercise routine week after week that provides the payoff you won't need to measure with a scale!

In short, use the scale to navigate your weight loss journey. Don't allow it to drive you off a cliff.

I welcome your feedback, questions, comments, and experiences. Please share at Donna@StopBeingFat101.com.

12

Learning to Exercise

Exercise creates a positive feeling that helps you stick with your weight loss goals.

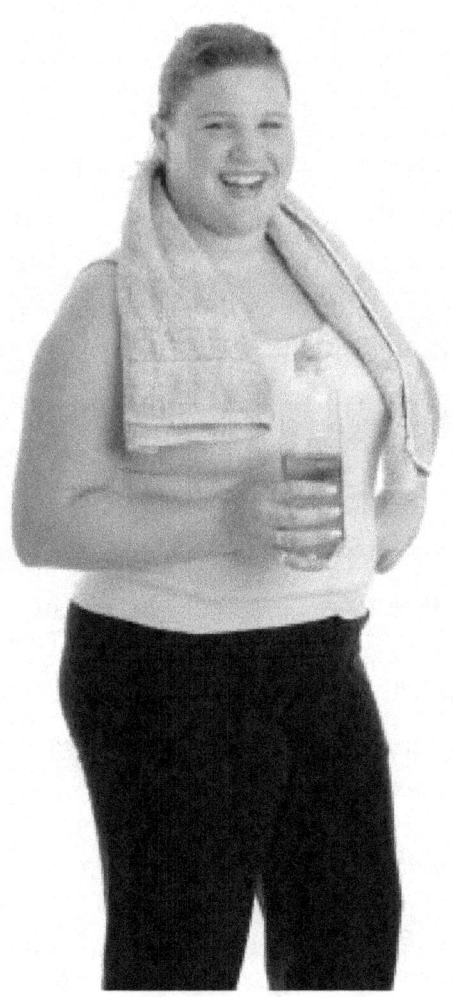

In all honesty, losing and maintaining a weight loss is 80–90% about what you eat. You can't undo 23 hours of overeating with 1 hour of exercise. Why then so much emphasis on exercise? Even those who proclaim to LIKE exercise, will admit that it is more about liking the results than it is about liking the actual act of exercising – most exercise nuts would choose an hour at the pool or with a good book if the results were the same. Exercise has benefits, of course, that most people are aware of. But, exercise also carries a benefit that most people don't recognize, especially for those trying to lose weight. A good sweat leaves you with a sense of accomplishment. You've demanded more from your body than you thought it could give, and that creates a positive feeling of power and control. Who wants to undo an hour of hard work in one 15 minute stop at the local hamburger joint? When your workout leaves you with a positive feeling, you WANT to eat to support your workout, which in turn allows you to workout more, which makes you feel good and on and on it goes. Ask anyone who makes exercise a part of their lifestyle and they will eventually mention the good feeling that comes with regular exercise.   They frequently described the muscle fatigue that comes with exercise as "a good kind of sore."

One of the most important elements of our weight loss program at my gym is the Exercise Education component. The National Weight Control Registry – a research study gathering information from people who have successfully maintained a weight loss of 30 lbs or more for at least 1 year – reports that 90% of those successful people **exercise an average of 1 hour daily** to maintain their weight loss.

Unlike you would expect, however, "exercise education" does not include instruction on how to do a bicep curl or different techniques for working your abs. Our version of exercise education is in teaching out-of-shape individuals how proper exercise **feels** – how to achieve that positive feeling mentioned above. Let me explain with an example.

Let's say you are one of the 7 in 10 adult Americans who don't exercise enough and you are determined to start running. You set out through the neighborhood with your sweat band and iPod, wearing the new running shoes purchased to confirm your commitment to this resolution. Two blocks down the road, your legs start to ache. Doubt creeps in – is a mile first time out really a reasonable goal? Another block or two and your breathing is labored. You are gasping for air, lungs and throat burning as your body attempts to pull in enough oxygen. When you stop – give up, that is – before you've reached the half mile mark, everything aches, you are panting, and you feel nauseous. Beaten, you begin the walk home, wondering if you will ever reach a point when a mile becomes possible.

What makes fit people different? Even a marathon runner reaches a point somewhere on the 26 mile journey where her legs ache, her throat burns and she feels like vomiting, just as you did on your first run. It takes her much longer to get to that point, but the fact is her first steps toward running a marathon started just as your first run started. The difference is that she has come to learn that exercise is more mental than physical. She pushes herself to the point where it becomes physically uncomfortable. Then her mental strength kicks in to push a tiny bit further, not just the first time, not just for races, but **every time she runs.** Simply put, her workout begins where your workout has ended. She can't help but increase her endurance and fitness level – she increases both every time she runs.

Everyone knows the value of regular exercise. We know it's important to your health, quality of life and emotional well–being. But, let's be honest – we only care that it makes us look and feel better, right? We focus on the numerous physical benefits of regular exercise, but learning to exercise is as much about training your mind as it is about training your body. So, lace up your shoes, go to the pool, get to the gym, but do whatever it takes to make exercise a part of your weight loss program. You will be amazed at the difference just a couple weeks will make when you commit to regular exercise.

I welcome your feedback, questions, comments, and experiences. Please share at Donna@StopBeingFat101.com.

13

Getting Started

Starting an exercise program is easy. Sticking with it is the challenge!

I started exercising regularly when I was 11 years old. That is 43 years – 43 sweaty years
of smelly socks, sore muscles and the inevitable wedgie that comes with kicking,
stretching, and generally forcing my body into contorted positions resembling the twisted shape of a paper clip. I could pretend to know the magic formula that will inspire you to start and stick with an exercise routine, but frankly, I don't recall how I did it myself. Oh, sure, I was an overweight kid, desperate to lose weight and feel like one of the group (rather than the ENTIRE group), but what ultimately motivated me to adopt a regular routine, I can't say. Exercising has become part of who I am, as much a part of me as my brown eyes and quirky sense of humor. Too many years have passed. And, as my kids are fond of pointing out, "you don't need sweating with the oldies, Mom, you ARE an Oldie!"

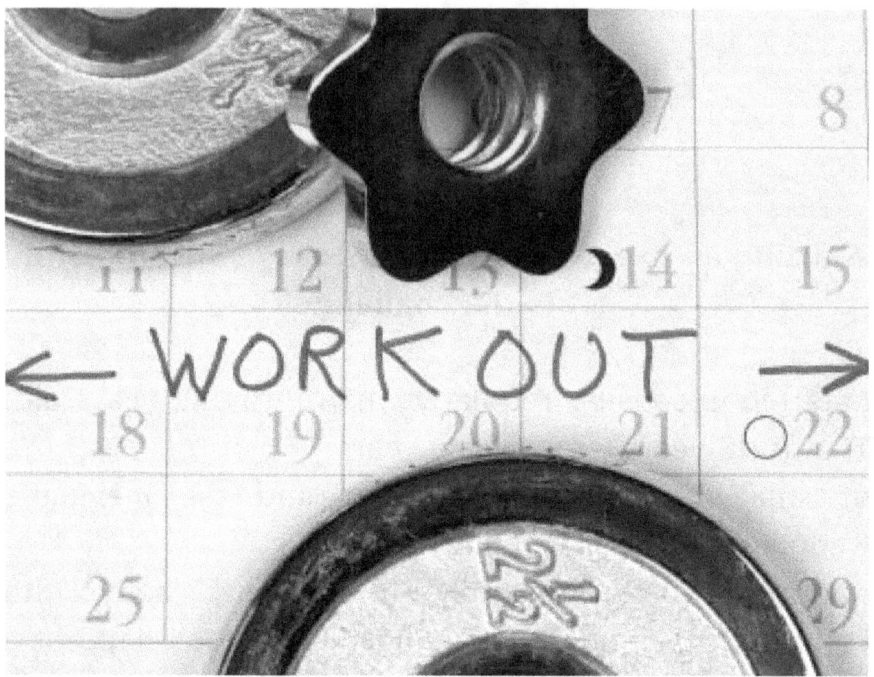

What I can give you is some practical advice – pitfalls to watch out for, how to avoid setting yourself up for failure. In the end, however, the only person who dictates your success is you. YOU will have to do the work and make the commitment to exercise. And, even though you might hope for the foolproof secret to success, you know deep down it is simply hard work that will get the job done.

I've always contended that the hardest part of any exercise routine is not the exercise, but the routine. Doing those sit-ups, push-ups and leg lifts is easy compared to overpowering the part of you that would much rather open a bag of chips and pop a disk in the DVD player. So, when you are ready to tackle your evil twin, the lazy slug, be certain you are mentally prepared. Look at your upcoming calendar and pick two consecutive weeks that look relatively free – no dinners with visiting dignitaries or nights on the town with touring rock bands. Block off those weeks and plan to keep them open. Don't fool yourself into thinking that you would be better off trying to offset a week of parties by attempting to start an exercise program the same week. Unless someone has perfected aerobic eating, it is not likely you will find the time for both activities. As much as humanly possible, attempt to exercise every day of that two weeks, even if it is just a 15-minute walk around the neighborhood. Don't think past the two weeks. Even if you fall right back into your indulge and bulge habits, you will have proven to yourself that you can succeed at exercising. I started and stopped exercising several times before it became part of my lifestyle. Each time I learned a little more about my own motivation. Each time it became a little easier to get started again.

Once you have established the exercise habit, pick a workout you can stick with. Try several activities. Never pick a workout simply because it burns the most calories, is the latest trend, or will impress your friends. Pick something that appeals to some part of you. Many runners will tell you that it is being outdoors, pounding the pavement with only their thoughts and their iPod to keep them company that motivates them to continue running. Personally, I put running on my list of LEAST favorite things to do, just after getting a root canal. My workout of choice is TaeRobics®. For me it is the constantly changing routine, the motivation that comes from exercising with a group and the social aspect – the people I workout with have become my friends. One "size" does NOT fit all when it comes to exercise, so take the time to shop for your "size".

When first beginning an exercise program, have a backup plan in the event you miss your regular workout. As challenging as it is to establish the habit of exercise, dropping the habit is as easy as finding a pornographic website on the Internet….uh, well, so I'm told. If you miss your 6 PM TaeRobics® class on Wednesday, go for a walk on your lunch hour on Thursday. It isn't important that you match the intensity of your regular workout or even the time spent doing it. What is important is keeping the habit. As you exercise, week after week, year after year, you will find that family, your job and other responsibilities and opportunities will force you to alter your exercise routine as well as the time you choose to enjoy it. When I first started exercising, I had to fight the temptation to skip my routine. When it became a habit, missing a routine made me anxious – convinced that I was back on the path to my former slovenly ways. Now that exercise is part of my lifestyle, I can miss a routine here and there with no guilt or concern about "making it up". Exercise has become as natural as sleeping. When I have a late night and don't get enough sleep, I never worry that I won't be able to catch up on sleep the next night.

"If it is important enough, you will find the time." How many of us have cringed at those
words while thinking "and here I've been wasting that hour between 3 and 4 AM!" The
statement is true, to some extent, but it is an over-simplification of the 24-hour challenge we all face. Exercise is important to me so I do find time for it. But, not without giving up other activities I wish I had time for. I would love to read more often, but I don't have the time. I would like to keep my house cleaner, but I don't have the time. I would like to take up painting again, but I don't have the time (a big relief to anyone with taste). The fact is we all have activities, habits or hobbies that are non-negotiable to us – a part of our lifestyle that we will not give up. The trick is to identify those activities that are non-negotiable to YOU. By doing that, you've determined, by default, those activities you are willing to give up, willing to replace with regular exercise. This is tough to do, but vitally important if you want to succeed in establishing an exercise routine. Let's face it, with the possible exception of the Maytag® repairman, no one I know has an hour of time every other day just waiting to be filled with exercise.

Hopefully, I've offered enough ideas to get you started, enough strategies to make you optimistic about your chances for success. We all know that regular exercise is important to your health, quality of life, emotional well being, and blah, blah, blah – well you've all heard that lecture. Go ahead and admit it, though – you secretly suspect that exercise and healthy eating doesn't really make you live longer....it just SEEMS longer, right? Be prepared for a pleasant surprise. Once you've made exercise part of your lifestyle, you will find that you workout not just because of the way it makes you feel, but because working out is so damn much fun! Here's to your success!

I welcome your feedback, questions, comments, and experiences. Please share at
Donna@StopBeingFat101.com.

14

The Best Diet is the One You Will Follow

Sorry to disappoint, but I really DON'T have a diet book I am trying to sell!

I will admit it, I have great abs – it is what I am known for at the gym Partly this is because my body type just doesn't carry weight around the middle, so there IS a genetic component to it. However, 90% of what gives me my "trademark abs" I owe directly to my diet. There isn't a drop in the gene pool that can make up for a high body fat percentage or a poor diet. Still, I have the following conversation with clients on a regular basis...

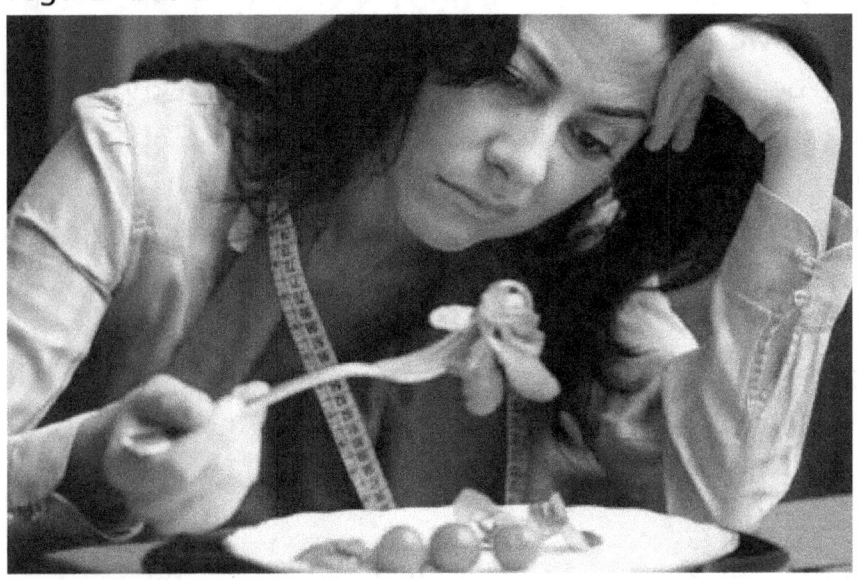

Client: How do I get abs like yours?

Me: It's really about body fat percentage.

Client: Do you work your abs every day?

Me: It's true that I work out hard, but mostly it's just diet.

Client: Is it crunches or do you do something special?

Me: You have good abs, too, or you wouldn't be able to sit up. You just need to lose the fat covering them.

Client: You must do a lot of twisting exercises.

Aaaargh!!!!

Diet is king in weight loss – you MUST take in fewer calories than you burn. Beyond that it needs to be a well-balanced diet that provides you with enough protein, carbs and fat to fuel your workouts, along with other essential vitamins, minerals and nutrients your body needs. Too often people get hung up on the teeny weeny details of what they should and should not be eating. Is the white meat on a chicken better than the dark? Should potatoes be avoided? Is peanut butter okay or should it be almond butter? To obsess over the HEALTHIEST choice in a diet seems peculiar when you are carrying 80 extra pounds around. If you are fat, it's extremely likely that you've tried one or more diets to lose weight – you already KNOW what you should be eating. However, a few guidelines might be helpful for those who have not.

Eat breakfast – this gets your metabolism started.

Stay away from processed foods – you are better off sticking with fresh foods.

Stay away from restaurants – you have no control over what goes in a restaurant meal.

Stick with scheduled meal times – don't eat impulsively. PLAN (there is that word again!) to eat every 2-3 hours, 250 – 300 calories. If it is not time for a scheduled meal, DO NOT EAT. Mealtime is not when you stop at the gas station and your favorite snack is on sale at the register. Mealtime is not when you go to the movie theater and the concession stand has fresh popcorn. Smaller, more frequent meals keep your metabolism cranking. Until this became a habit for me, I set up daily reminders in my electronic calendar to go off at the same times daily to remind me to eat.

Learn to distinguish between food and fun. Society has turned food into entertainment. Have a birthday, and someone bakes a cake. Gather with your buddies to play poker, and everyone pitches in for pizza. Plan a get together with your girlfriends and the first requirement is picking the restaurant where you will meet. Food is what your body requires. Fun is burgers, fries, pizza, cookies, chips, etc.

Drink LOTS of water, 8 glasses or more daily. Your liver metabolizes fat and it requires plenty of water to function properly.

Do not drink alcohol. This is a killer for many people who reason that if they include alcohol calories into their calorie count for the day, they should be able to enjoy a beer or a glass of wine. In addition, it is widely known that moderate amounts of alcohol can lower the risk of heart disease and increase the levels of "good cholesterol." Personally, I see no harm with most things – in moderation – for individuals who are living a healthy lifestyle. The key part of that last sentence, however, is **healthy lifestyle.** Alcohol has no place in a weight loss regimen for many reasons.

First off, alcohol is empty calories. There are many foods which you will never see on any sensible weight loss plan that still have some nutritional value – not so with alcohol. Alcohol lowers blood sugar levels. This leaves you feeling hungry, a recipe for overeating. Alcohol also dehydrates the drinker. I've already discussed the importance of staying properly hydrated. And, despite the drowsy relaxed, feeling that usually accompanies its consumption, alcohol has been shown to actually disrupt sleep. Proper rest is another key element in weight loss.

But, here's the kicker... according to the Mayo Clinic®, **alcohol inhibits fat loss**. I could provide the scientific explanation for this, but here is the short version: your body metabolizes alcohol differently than it metabolizes fat and carbs. When you put alcohol in, your body begins working to eliminate it from your system immediately, and the processing of food becomes secondary. This leads to food being stored and synthesized as fat, which can lead to weight gain. The evidence is clear that moderate alcohol consumption does carry health benefits. But, a healthy lifestyle produces similar results without the hangover.

When I lost 85+ pounds 35 years ago, I followed a very well known program that is popular still today. It was a structured program that defined, rather rigidly, the type and amounts of food I needed to eat. At that point in my life, it was exactly what I needed. The key phrase is at that point in my life. This program has evolved over the years and is drastically different than the program I followed 35 years ago. However, if I were to find myself in a position where I needed to lose 20-30 pounds, I would NEVER use the "new and improved" program. It's a good program that many people love, but it is TOO flexible for me! I am overwhelmed by too many variables when I am trying to lose weight. With my busy life, I need structure. I need to eliminate some of the decision-making. In fact, **I wouldn't even use the old version of the program that I succeeded with 35 years ago.** I learned a great deal about healthy eating and about my own culinary likes and dislikes from that diet, but it just doesn't fit my lifestyle these days. As I said before, it is not at all important to find a diet that "works for you" but a diet you can work with.

There you have it – a "diet" to live by! Many of you will still be frustrated that I won't tell you exactly what you need to eat. I'm not a nutritionist, so I'm not even qualified to do that. The fact is, we have fat nutritionists in our Stop Being Fat Network program all the time, so clearly it is not about information. On the rare occasion when I've agreed to write down my typical diet for a client, the client always admits to modifying based on her likes and dislikes.

Use common sense and count calories. Ultimately, the best diet is the one that you will follow.

I welcome your feedback, questions, comments, and experiences. Please share at
Donna@StopBeingFat101.com.

15

My #1 Weight Loss Tip

It's not a specific diet or particular exercise that makes the difference.

At the age of 54, I am in the best shape of my life (except for a few pesky gray hairs!) Needless to say, most people are shocked to learn that I struggled with weight issues as a child, and weighed over 200 lbs at 19 years old. It follows that, over the course of our weight loss program at the gym, inevitably someone asks, "What is YOUR diet like on a day to day basis?"

These people are more than just curious. They are struggling with the very challenges I faced 30+ years ago and continue to face to this day. They believe I have somehow found the perfect solution, and it's human nature to hope they can make it work for themselves as well. It's true that I eat a very balanced, healthy diet. But, my "secret" is not the diet I choose. After all, **every** diet will help you lose weight...if you follow it!

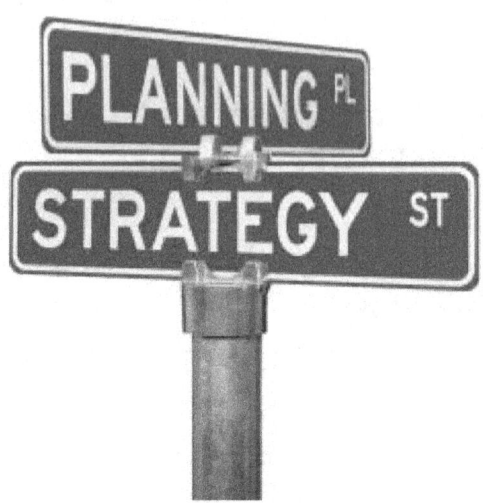

If I could pick one thing that makes the difference for me between a day of healthy living and a day of poor choices, that thing would be **PREPARATION!** It requires more than good intentions to get thru a day when you have embarked on a weight loss regimen. Good intentions go out the window the minute you need to work late, the car breaks down or the dog gets sick. Every weekend, I try to spend 2-3 hours preparing for the next week. I peel carrots, prepare soup, steam brown rice, cook oatmeal – whatever it takes to get thru the week with plenty of good eating options at my fingertips. That doesn't mean that I plan every meal to the mouthful for my week ahead. But, I know that I will never arrive home tired and hungry at 9pm, to find a pantry full of nothing but junk food and snacks.

You may think you are a prepared dieter as well, yet still find there are times when the poor choice is the easier choice. This is rarely true in my life - I have given the word "preparation" a whole new meaning! For example, if we both like grapes, we might both purchase a pound or two at the start of the week. Chances are, you now consider yourself prepared with a healthy snack on hand. I'm going to take it one step further, however. I will take my pound of grapes, rinse them off, and place them in the fridge in plastic baggies full of single size servings. The poor choice still wins out occasionally, even when there is an army of bagged grapes lined up on the bottom shelf of the fridge. But, there is **no** excuse that allows me to forgive choosing potato chips over rinsed, measured, ready-to-eat grapes. That's accountability!

Being prepared to eat right applies to more than just having healthy food ready and available. As you might imagine, I always have my meals and snacks for the day with me. That's true even when I have lunch plans. Yep, that's right - **even when I have lunch plans.** We all have busy lives. Just as I've had to cancel appointments and reschedule meetings, there is no predicting when my lunch companion may have to do the same. It's surprising how often I need my backup lunch. And, if I don't need it, it goes into the fridge and I am ready for the next day.

Being prepared for my workout is also part of the daily plan. I pack my gym bag the night before and place it by the door to grab on the way out. And, just like my backup lunch, even if I have plans that interfere with my workout, the bag still goes with me. Plans change, all the time! I also bring my workout clothes with me on every vacation I take. I don't obsess about working out on vacation – vacations are for relaxing, even for a gym rat. But, if I have some down time or the mood strikes, I am ready to work out.

Preparation. That's my key. Not just preparation for the day I have planned, but preparation for the surprises that the day may bring. You can't plan for every contingency, to be sure. But, trust me when I say weight loss **never** occurs without a plan.

I welcome your feedback, questions, comments, and experiences. Please share at
Donna@StopBeingFat101.com.

16

More Weight Loss Tips

Keep in mind...you didn't get fat by eating when you were hungry, you became fat by eating when you were NOT hungry.

In the last chapter, I discussed my Number One weight loss tip: Preparation. For most people, preparation is going to be the key to successful weight loss. HOPING the day falls into place to make healthy choices possible is not the way to go. Assuming you've already conquered the preparation piece of it, there will still be numerous challenges and temptations you will have to deal with and overcome if you are to be successful. These are going to be different for everyone. In this chapter, I've listed some challenges that I face. It's likely that at least one or two them are challenges for you as well and these hints will help you through the rough spots!

Tip: Never get in your car without a day's supply of healthy food choices. This is really an extension of my #1 tip, preparation overkill, if you will. If you started each day with a map of how you expected the day to unfold, nine times out of ten, there would be a surprise in your day. If you are already prepared, this is no more complicated than getting a small cooler and a re-freezeable ice pack to keep in the trunk.

Tip: Don't be afraid to bring your own snacks to a party or to a movie. This is self-explanatory. I have a friend who still tells people about the time we went to a movie theater and I pulled carrots and celery out of my pocket.

Tip: If you have favorite treats you just can't give up, freeze them and pull them out one at a time...it allows you to enjoy them without binging on them. One of my favorite treats is brownies – homemade or from the box, with or without icing, baked in the Ultimate Brownie Pan® or my beat up metal 9"x13" pan, I find them hard to resist. Rather than do without, I will bake a batch, cut them up, and toss them in the freezer. When I have a craving, I pull one out of the freezer and leave it to thaw. Once I've made the decision to treat myself, it no longer nags at my will power – the craving seems to go away. More often than not, I forget that there is a brownie sitting out, thawing on the counter. When I re-discover it, sometimes hours later, I can enjoy it and be satisfied without the nagging craving that might result in binge eating. There is a flaw with this tip...if your weakness is ice cream, this won't help you much!

Tip: If you are tempted, "ruin" your taste for food. This tip actually came from one of the guys in our Stop

Being Fat Network who successfully lost 30 lbs in 9 weeks. He bought a package of extremely strong mints in a flavor he didn't like. When he felt like eating something he shouldn't, he popped a mint instead. As he put it, "NOTHING tastes good after you've had one of those!"

Tip: If you think a party, gathering or event is going to tempt you, DON'T GO! I can hear you protesting now. How many invitations to lunch or a night out with the girls do you accept that could be skipped? When I figured out what was required to lose weight, and success became easy for me, I looked forward to each new day. I couldn't wait to get up and lose more weight! Truthfully, I didn't want to sabotage my success. I knew that I could party every week when I had reached my goal weight. Of course, there are some events that are just too special to miss – weddings, reunions and the like. A woman from our Stop Being Fat Network talked of how she opened a beer at a reunion, emptied it and filled it with tap water, pretending to drink all night long! She actually enjoyed pretending she was getting drunk, watching the antics of her girlfriends through sober eyes. Trust me....when you step on the scale and see your goal weight, you will not say, "Yeah, I look and feel great, but I sure wish I'd had that pizza on February 28th.

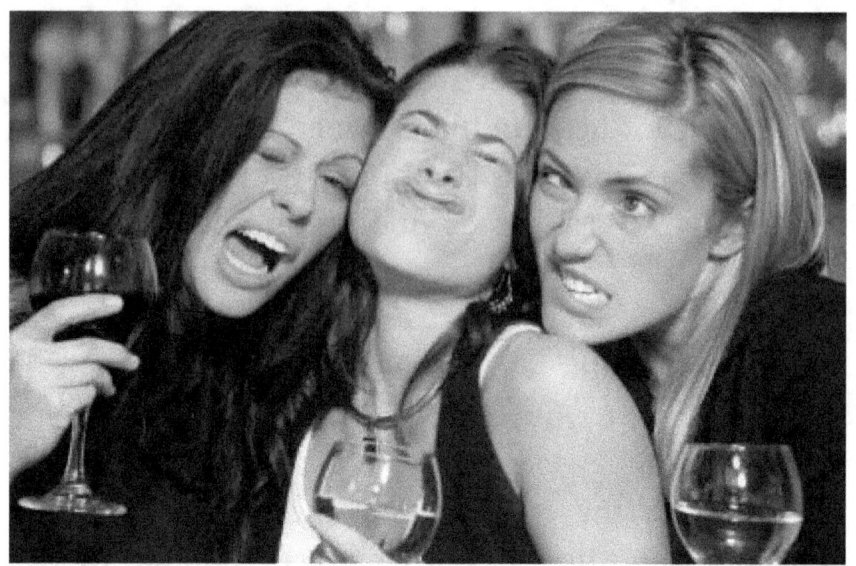

These are just a few of my "Tips to Lose By." We all face different challenges – these may help you with your healthy lifestyle demons or they may not! If you would like to share your weight loss tips, I would love to hear them! Email them to me at Donna@StopBeingFat101.com, subject Stop Being Fat Lifestyle Tips. Thanks!

I welcome your feedback, questions, comments, and experiences. Please share at Donna@StopBeingFat101.com.

17

Choose Your Mood

Many occasions and events are challenging for dieters, but the holidays present a particularly difficult challenge.

It starts with October and that familiar feel of Fall in the air. Mornings are cooler, evenings are "nippy". The wind picks up during the days, and you hide under increasingly bulky clothes. Soon it's Halloween. You hustle your tired little trick-or-treaters off to bed – then you go through their Halloween "stash" and pull out all the Snickers!® "A couple candy bars won't hurt," you reason. Repeat as often as needed over the next several days as you polish off the candy you DIDN'T give out to the ghosts and goblins that showed up on your own doorstep that Halloween night. Just about the time Walgreens® stops selling Halloween candy at 75% off (well, you'd be an idiot to turn THAT down – they are practically giving it away!), Thanksgiving comes calling. Ah, Turkey Day!...when the bird gets stuffed, and so do you! And, we all know the best part about Thanksgiving, right? The leftovers! When you aren't making a mashed potato, stuffing, and gravy sandwich, you are "getting out of the kitchen" at your favorite local restaurant. The holidays roll on toward Christmas – an endless blizzard of goodies received, parties to attend, holiday lunches, home baked gifts and on and on. You snap out of your sugar coma around December 27th, clothing dusted with the crumbs of Christmas cookies, wondering where you left your waistline. No point in starting a diet now – the New Year's Eve Party is only a few days away. By the time January 1st dawns, you are depressed, moody, several pounds heavier and not particularly amused that your best friend remembers your New Year's resolution to lose weight. SOUND FAMILIAR????

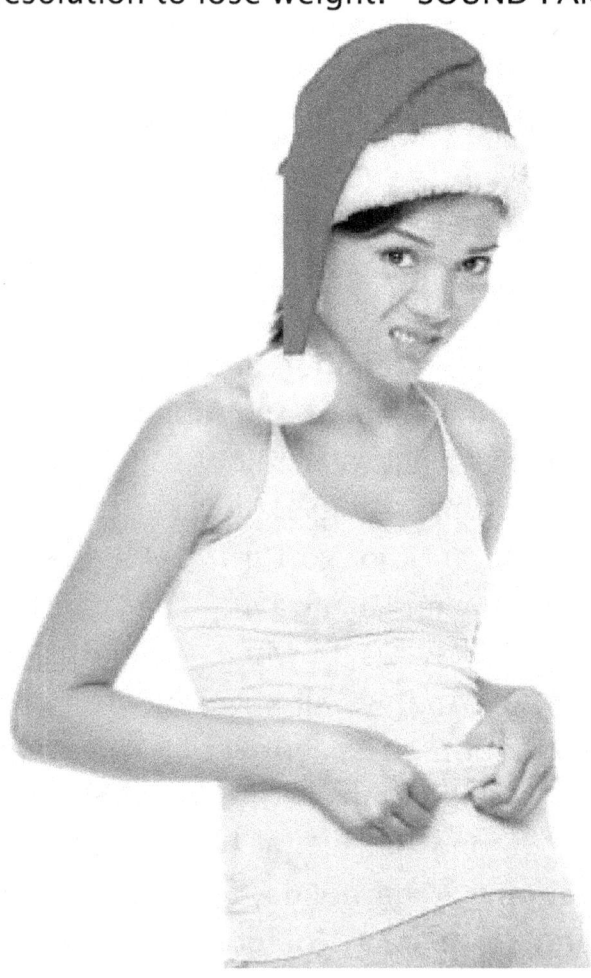

It's no surprise that the average person gains 3 to 7 pounds every holiday season, and, that's the average person. If you are an...um, shall we say "overachiever", you can pack on quite a few more pounds than that. Fast forward to January 1st and think about how you will feel – your mood and emotional state – if you are the "average" person. Most people fall into one of two categories. First, there is the person for whom the holidays were a disappointment. Maybe it was the stress of the countless holiday obligations. Maybe it was the tedious task of spending what should be the best time of year with relatives that make the Osbourne's® look like The Partridge Family®. Or, maybe it was as simple as not getting what you wanted, whether that was a holiday bonus or a little quality time with your kids. Regardless of the reason, somehow the holiday did not meet your expectations. The second type of person had a GREAT holiday. It was partying, seeing friends, gift exchanges, days off work and the many fun things to do that come with the holidays. Regardless of which type person you are, January 1st arrives with the following constants: it's cold; it's dreary; the bills are here; you won't see another day off until Martin Luther King Day, or maybe Good Friday, or, yikes!!...maybe not even till Memorial Day! Pack on several extra pounds, and NOW how is your mood? You are not only depressed and gloomy, you feel bad about yourself.

Admit it. Every January 1st as you plan your grocery list for the diet you are about to start, you resolve that next year things will be different...that next year you will not let your holiday eating get so out of control. Well, guess what? Next year is here. The time is now.

LET'S MAKE THIS HOLIDAY SEASON DIFFERENT!!!!

Take charge and choose your mood for January 1st. You know what it feels like to be depressed and not happy with yourself, we've all been there. This winter, break with tradition and arrive on the other side of December slimmer, healthier, and with the positive and determined attitude that comes from succeeding at the challenging task of losing weight.

Diet over the holidays???? Why that's absolutely crazy, right? Before you have me committed, however, consider the following:

- ☒ NO ONE gains 7 pounds by eating one slice of pecan pie, or one holiday dinner – its what you do the ENTIRE holiday season!
- ☒ if the fun of a party was about the food, you could have a blast every weekend by preparing a large buffet and eating alone in front of the TV
- ☒ no one ever got arrested for baking a sweet potato casserole or Christmas cookies in July, so

you really don't have to eat as much as you can consume "while it's there"

- [x] gyms are a lot less crowded over the holidays
- [x] the seventeenth piece of fudge really does taste just like the first
- [x] unless Aunt Esther does her knitting in the next office, she won't be hurt by finding out that you brought her gift of candied almonds in to share with your co-workers
- [x] cleaning up at the after holiday sales is a lot more fun when you are NOT buying clothes in a larger size

Simply put, there is no time like the present. Personally, I've never made a New Year's Resolution....never. If I want to make a positive change in my life, I plan how to approach it and I execute the plan. Have I ever failed? Sure! But, not limiting myself to "the first day of the New Year" allows me to plug away through the ups and downs, restart and rediscover my motivation as many times as necessary until I get it right and make the lifestyle change I desire. Why set yourself up for failure? There is nothing magical about January 1st that makes it easier to diet and lose weight – if anything, the post-holiday gloom and depression make it more difficult.

If you are <u>truly</u> ready to make the lifestyle change and lose those unhealthy excess pounds, NOW is the time.

Losing weight is a challenge that will NOT be any easier after January 1st than it will be before January 1st – trust me.   Don't look ahead to the New Year. Make **this** year different.   Choose better health as your holiday gift to yourself!

I welcome your feedback, questions, comments, and experiences. Please share at Donna@StopBeingFat101.com.

18

Are You an Expert?

It is easy to recognize an expert at being thin.

I've trained with a 6th degree black belt and former international karate competitor for some time now. Prior to that, I trained for several years at a local martial arts school. While I liked the owners and students at the local school, and the workout was challenging, it didn't take more than a few weeks of training with my current instructor to realize I was dealing with a totally different standard. He is an "old school" instructor – training is as much about skill, discipline, and proper technique as it is about learning the simple mechanics.

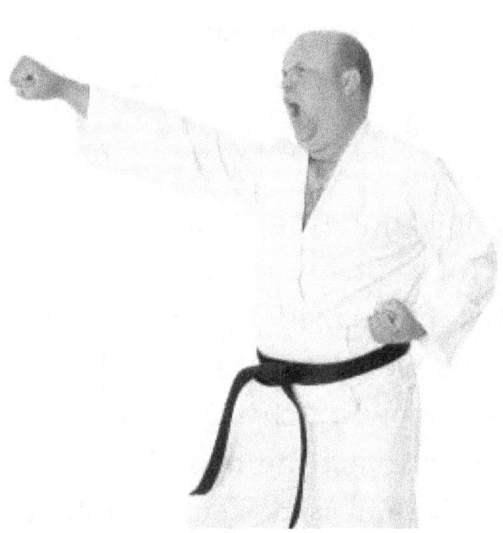

When you visit a karate class, you will find the instructor addressing rows of students all dressed in their "gis" or traditional karate uniform. At a glance, the students all look the same. Soon you notice the pecking order. The black, brown and higher belt ranks stand in the front row; the newest students, white belts, stand in the back. Intermediate belts line up in-between. This arrangement is as true in the old standard, as it is in the new standard. The difference with the old standard was that a black belt actually **meant** something. It signified an elite level of skill, training, and discipline that was earned and worn with pride. Nowadays, a black belt indicates nothing more than a student who has memorized enough techniques and paid enough money. To be certain, there are schools which still operate under the old standard, as there are still students in new standard schools who set their own bar and strive for a higher level of skill. But, it is fairly easy nowadays for a karate black belt to masquerade as an expert – there are just too many schools which allow it.

This is simply not true with weight loss and fitness. When the topic of my occupation comes up in social situations, I'm amazed by the number of fat, out of shape people who launch into a litany of how healthy they eat and how much they work out. I simply nod politely and interject the occasional "is that so?" After all, if an individual is perfectly content with herself, it doesn't bother or concern me in the least. Just like today's karate black belt, however, she is masquerading as an expert. Unlike today's karate black belt, she can't hide the deception by dressing a certain way or by standing in the front row.

How can you tell a friend has a new hair cut? You notice her new style. How can you tell she also got a manicure at the salon? Her nails are trimmed, polished and look nice. If you switch on your own powers of observation one day, you can learn a LOT about total strangers you pass on the street or stand behind in line at the grocery. A man with a cast and crutches has injured a leg. A woman with a cigarette smell on her breath is a smoker. If you are fat, I know instantly that you are eating too much – all I have to do is look at you.

On the flip side, by looking at me, you should be able to tell that I work out regularly and eat no more than my body requires. As someone who was fat all through my childhood, adolescent, and teen years, I face special challenges. Obese youngsters often have more and bigger fat cells. Those fat cells do not "disappear". They shrunk as I lost weight, but without surgical intervention (as in liposuction) they will always be with me ready to absorb any fat that I eat, like a sponge with no limit. Yet, most fat people assume I am "lucky" – I must have a high metabolism, I must be naturally thin. Just last week I was having a discussion with one of the clients at the gym. She had signed up for a race that was taking place the following day. She did not want to do it, but to her credit, had committed to the race and was determined to follow through. I laughingly told her I would NEVER commit to a race as I hate running. "Yeah," she said, "but you are genetically gifted." This woman has seen me workout, sweat pouring off me, muscles giving out, not just now and then, but every time I work out, 5-6 times a week. Yeah, that's it - I'm genetically gifted. To assume that a good physique is the luck of the draw is an insult to me. It seems the harder I work the luckier I get!

When you take on the monumental task to change who you are, and take the difficult steps to build a lifestyle that supports your weight loss and fitness, it is easy to become discouraged when the fat does not drop off and the muscles don't bulge as quickly as you would like. The day will come, however, when you receive your first unsolicited compliment: "Hey, you've lost weight! Looking good!" Smile and enjoy it. It means you are at the front of the class achieving an A+ in your new field of study. You become an expert at being thin by actually being thin. There is no way to deceive anyone on this.

I welcome your feedback, questions, comments, and experiences. Please share at
Donna@StopBeingFat101.com.

19

The Fat Acceptance Movement

You can be fat, happy and self accepting, but you can't force others to accept it.

Every few weeks there is a news item, internet posting or magazine article about discrimination targeting the obese. We've even seen the emergence of fat activist groups, such as the Fat Acceptance Movement. I'm a strong believer that everyone has the right to be exactly who they want to be and if an individual is happy and secure as a fat person, it has nothing to do with me. While the goal of acceptance is a worthy one on any level, the fact is, no organization will ever be able to dictate opinion. Declaring a movement and demanding acceptance does not make it suddenly happen. Like it or not, no one ever comes to our weight loss program because they are happy with their weight. They come to me because they've seen the stares, they've heard the snickering, they've looked in a mirror and said, "I don't want to live this way anymore."

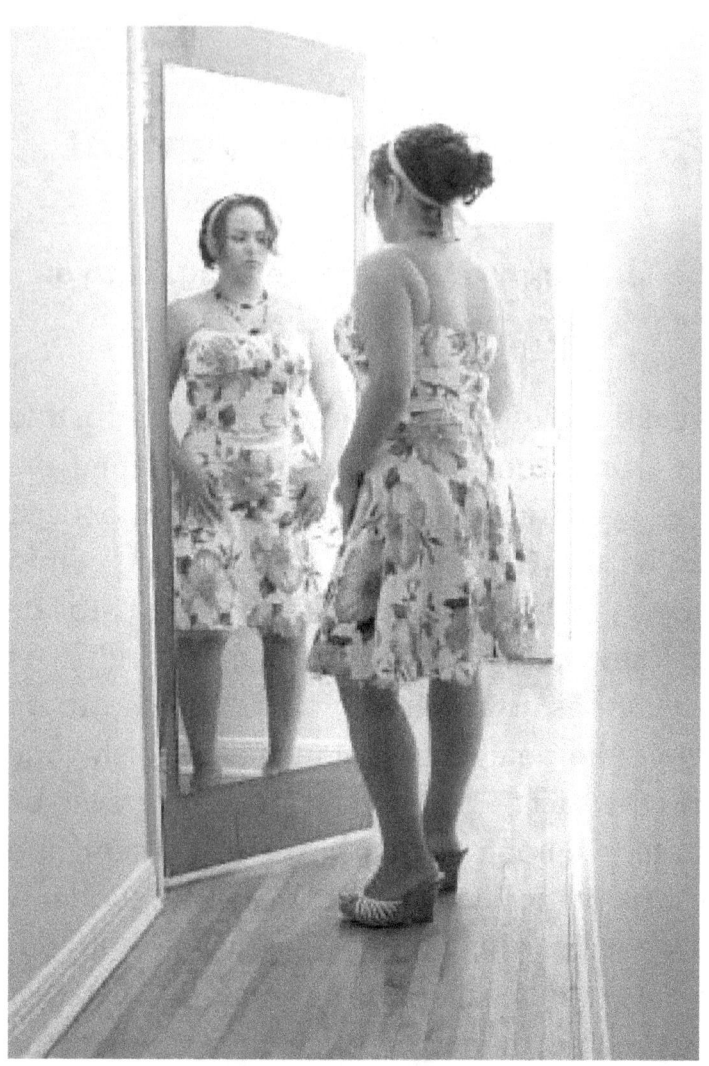

Fat activists will argue that fitness is not defined by a dress size. This is true enough. I've known many thin people who were completely unhealthy. Statistically speaking, however, there is a direct, measurable correlation between BMI and a number of chronic diseases, particularly diabetes. But, this is not really about fitness and health, is it? This is about self-esteem and honesty.

I've been on both sides of the "Fat Acceptance Movement." As a fat child and teenager, I endured the taunts of my peers as well as frequent embarrassing situations created by insensitive adults. It is as true today as it was then – fat kids are bullied and teased by their peers. In an effort to lose weight, I started exercising at the age of 11. By 19, I was the fittest fat person you would ever meet, far more fit than many of my skinny friends. No one cared about my fitness. My social life was defined by my fatness, despite our politically correct world which likes to pretend no one cares that you are fat.

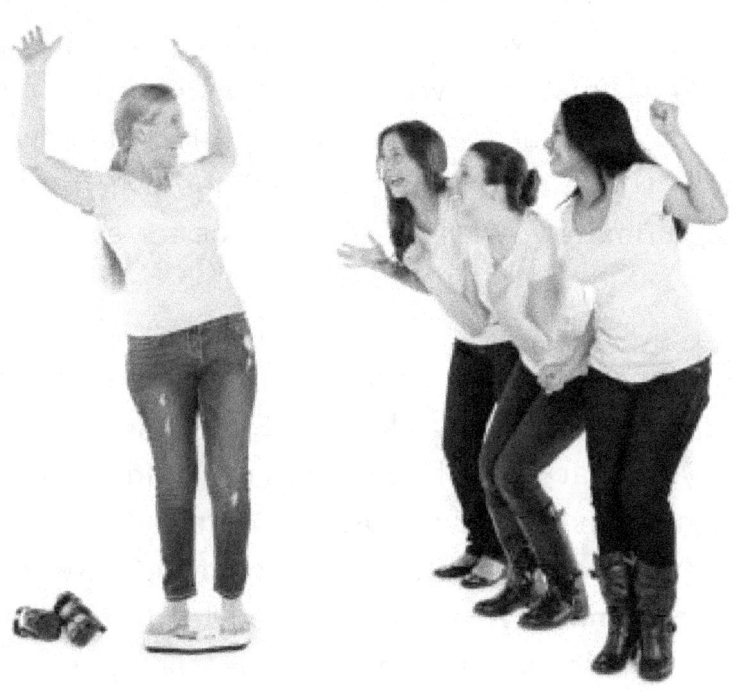

I saw an ad in the personals section of the newspaper recently which ended with the following statement, "Do not apply if you call yourself a BBW, curvy, big and beautiful or any other term that means fat." This is hurtful, but it IS reality. Years ago, I had a conversation with a good friend. He is, to this day, one of the most considerate people I know. At the time, he was struggling with some self-inflicted guilt. He was approaching an age when he wanted to settle down and start raising a family. He had many friends, a number of them girls, and a number of them interested in him. He confessed to me that try as he might, he simply could not find fat women attractive. This made him feel incredibly shallow and he didn't like it. I told him that attraction was 100% subjective and the only opinions which mattered were the opinions of the two people involved. I urged him to accept it as shallow if he must, but to attempt to force feelings which were not there, ultimately, was a waste of time for everyone involved.

If you are fat and happy with yourself, this does not apply to you. Carry on. It is not my intention to convince you that you should be thin. Unlike you, however, millions of fat people must care or weight loss would not be the multi-billion dollar industry that it is. I should not try to convince you to be thin any more than you should try to convince someone else that they must remain fat. If people care not to be fat, you cannot expect them to accept their fatness because you insist on it. This is not an argument. I am not on anyone's "side". For those who WANT to lose weight, my only job is to get them to accept the truth about how the process works.

To put it bluntly, there is no Fat Acceptance Movement. We all resent the fat traveler crowding us from the next plane seat and judge the fat mom buying lunch for her kids at a fast food restaurant. Men everywhere will admit to looking at the chubby women perched on barstools in a singles bar, and then moving on. This is a painful reality. It **IS** unjust to judge people by their appearance. Opinions can be based on ignorance, but they can't be dictated. If you are happy with yourself exactly as you are, thin or fat, carry on and more power to you! If, however, you are NOT happy about being judged for your size, the unfortunate reality is that you will have far more success changing yourself than changing the opinion of the world.

I welcome your feedback, questions, comments, and experiences. Please share at
Donna@StopBeingFat101.com.

20

So Now What?

For those who have made it to this page, I expect you've experienced a variety of emotions – amusement, anger, embarrassment, enlightenment and others.

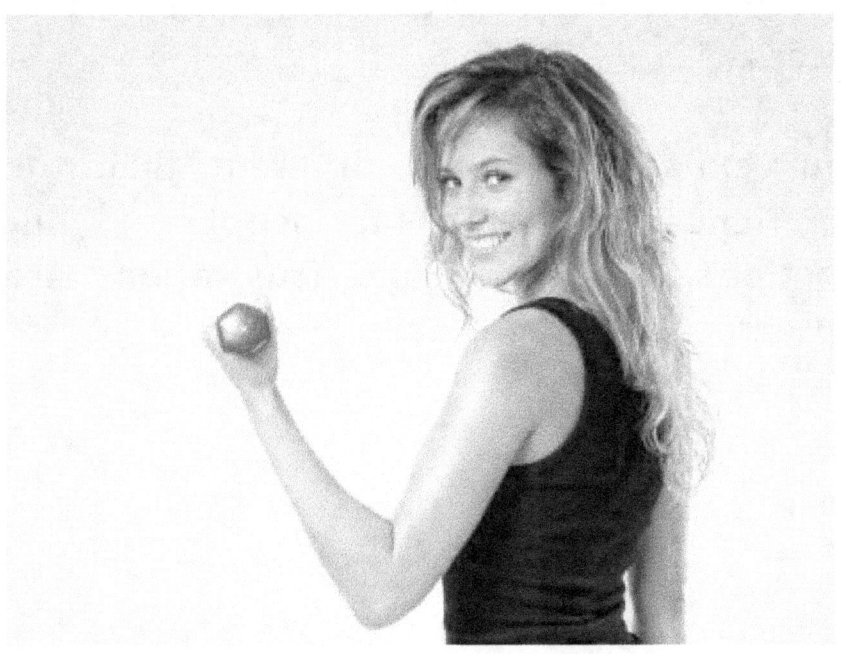

This is good. Rarely does lasting weight loss happen in individuals who put on a happy face, cover their emotions and pretend to be the jolly, carefree fat person. Even though the global obesity crisis has far reaching and insidious impact on our healthcare system, our workforce, and our society as a whole, it is unusual for a client seeking weight loss to come to us

STRICTLY for health reasons. The vast majority are here because their self esteem is suffering – they DON'T feel good about themselves or the way society views them.

If you learned nothing else from reading this book, I hope you have realized the following truths:

You really haven't "tried everything without success."

Your experience is no different than the experience of other fat people – your emotions, challenges and frustrations are quite normal and ordinary.

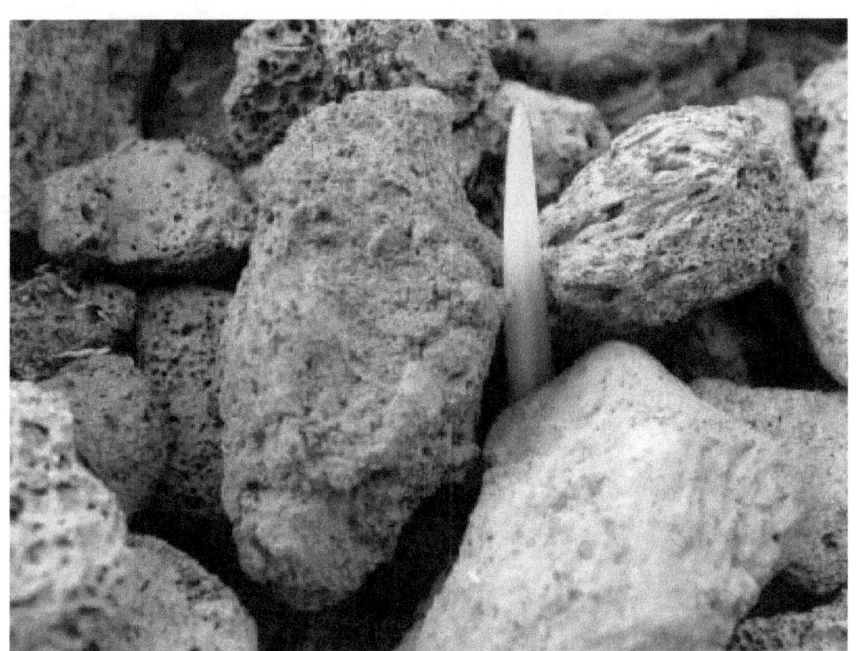

A lifetime of fitness and health does not just happen for people who are normal and ordinary. This is precisely why 90–95% of all people fail at permanent weight loss. If you want to lose weight AND keep the weight off, you must be an **extra**-ordinary person.

Expect it to be difficult. Expect setbacks. Expect resistance. Once you "get it", once you understand EXACTLY what it takes to lose weight, you will know it. You will feel powerful and in control, and weight loss will become effortless.

I welcome your feedback, questions, comments, and experiences. Please share at
Donna@StopBeingFat101.com.

STOP BEING FAT!

Yes! It's a choice!

Published by:

SanCo Media
www.SanCoMedia.com